EMQs in
SURGERY

EMQs in
SURGERY

Second edition

Mr Irfan Syed BSc(Hons) MBBS MRCS DO-HNS PGCertMedEd
Specialist Registrar ENT Surgery, Great Ormond Street Hospital,
London, UK

Mohammed Keshtgar BSc MBBS FRCSI FRCS(Gen) PhD
Consultant Surgical Oncologist, Royal Free Hampstead Foundation Trust;
Reader in Cancer Surgery, University College, London, UK

 CRC Press
Taylor & Francis Group
Boca Raton London New York

CRC Press is an imprint of the
Taylor & Francis Group, an **informa** business

First published in Great Britain as EMQs and Data Interpretation Questions in Surgery in 2008
This second edition published in 2013 by
CRC Press
Taylor & Francis Group
6000 Broken Sound Parkway NW, Suite 300
Boca Raton, FL 33487-2742

© 2013 by Taylor & Francis Group, LLC
CRC Press is an imprint of Taylor & Francis Group, an Informa business

No claim to original U.S. Government works

ISBN 13: 978-1-4441-6921-8 (pbk)
Version Date: 20120813

Visit the Taylor & Francis Web site at
http://www.taylorandfrancis.com

and the CRC Press Web site at
http://www.crcpress.com

Dedication

To Mum & Dad, Reshma and Zishan for their continued support.

To my wife Reshma for always being there.
Irfan Syed

Contents

Contributors

Mr Obiekezie Agu MS FRCS(Gen)
Consultant Vascular Surgeon, University College Hospital, London, UK

Miss Sarvi Banisadr BSc(Hons) MBBS MRCS
Specialist Registrar General Surgery, Watford General Hospital, UK

Mr Andrew Bath BMedSci BMBS FRCS(ORL)
Consultant ENT Surgeon, Norfolk and Norwich University Hospital, UK

Dr Pervinder Bhogal BSc (Hons), MBBS MRCS PGDipMedEd FRCR
Specialist Registrar Radiology, London Deanery, UK

Dr Brigitta Brandner FRCA MD
Consultant Anaesthetist, University College Hospital, London, UK

Mr Raymond Brown MA MBChir FRCS FRCOphth
Consultant Ophthalmologist, University Hospital of North Staffordshire, UK

Mr Fares Haddad BSc MCh(Orth) FRCS(Orth)
Consultant Orthopaedic Surgeon and Honorary Senior Lecturer,
University College London Hospitals, UK

Mr Naveed Jallali BSc MBChB(Hons) MRCS
Specialist Registrar, Plastic and Reconstructive Surgery, Royal Free Hospital,
London, UK

Mr Rohan Nauth-Misir BSc FRCS(Urol)
Consultant Urologist and Clinical Director Urology, University College Hospital,
London, UK

Dr Reshma Syed MBBS, MRCS(Ophth) MRCGP DRCOG DFSRH
GPwSI Ophthalmology, West Kent Primary Care Trust, Kent, UK

Dr Zishan Syed MB BChir MA MDCH
GPST2 Trainee, Kent, Surrey & Sussex Deanery, UK

Mr Peter Tassone MBChB MRCS
Specialist Registrar, ENT surgery, Norfolk and Norwich University Hospital, UK

Dr Patrick Wong FRCA
Consultant Anaesthetist, St George's Hospital, Tooting, London, UK

Preface

EMQs in Surgery, 2nd Edition has two main roles. First, we aim to provide a bank of questions for examination practice, as familiarity breeds confidence. The EMQ revision boxes in EMQs in Clinical Medicine, 2nd Edition (Hodder Arnold: 2011) have been popular and so we have included a separate revision boxes section for easy reference.

Second, we wanted to provide an informative text with detailed explanations, taking advantage of the collective knowledge from our colleagues in the surgical specialties.

We sincerely hope that this book helps you in the build-up to your examination and we wish you all the best in your medical career!

Irfan Syed and Mohammed Keshtgar

Acknowledgements

This book would not have been possible without the excellent work in reviewing and editing questions by our colleagues.

Many thanks to Jo Koster, Stephen Clausard and all the team at Hodder Arnold for their efforts in bringing this project to fruition.

SECTION 1: GENERAL SURGERY

QUESTIONS

1 The acute abdomen

A	acute porphyria	H	colorectal carcinoma
B	acute pancreatitis	I	diverticulosis
C	perforated viscus	J	duodenal ulcer
D	appendicitis	K	renal colic
E	small bowel obstruction	L	aortic dissection
F	acute cholecystitis	M	oesophageal atresia
G	large bowel obstruction			

For each clinical scenario below give the most likely cause for the clinical findings. Each option may be used only once.

1   A 36-year-old man complains of waves of pain in the lower left flank.

2   A 45-year-old man presents in A&E with severe epigastric pain radiating to the back and vomiting. On examination he is tachycardic with low blood pressure and respiratory distress. Past medical history includes gallstones and reflux oesophagitis.

3   A 44-year-old obese woman presents with continuous right upper quadrant pain, vomiting and fever. There is marked right upper quadrant tenderness when palpating on inspiration.

4   A 57-year-old man is brought to the emergency department complaining of severe generalized abdominal pain. On examination he looks systemically unwell and has a rigid abdomen. His wife reports a long history of intermittent epigastric pain after meals.

5   A 10-year-old boy presents with fever, nausea and right iliac fossa pain.

ANSWERS: see page 34

2 Chronic abdominal pain

A	biliary colic	H	Crohn's disease
B	gastric carcinoma	I	carcinoma of caecum
C	umbilical hernia	J	irritable bowel syndrome
D	primary sclerosing cholangitis	K	appendicitis
E	reflux oesophagitis	L	hepatocellular carcinoma
F	small bowel obstruction	M	diverticulitis
G	ulcerative colitis			

For each clinical scenario below give the most likely cause for the clinical findings. Each option may be used only once.

1   A 35-year-old man presents with weight loss, diarrhoea and abdominal pain. On examination he has aphthous ulcers in the mouth and a mass is palpable in the right iliac fossa. Blood tests reveal low serum B_{12} and folate.

2   A 26-year-old male presents with recurrent burning pain in the upper abdomen and chest following meals. He is otherwise well.

3   A 21-year-old student presents with a several month history of bloating and diffuse abdominal pain associated with alternating constipation and diarrhoea. Colonoscopy and inflammatory markers are normal.

4   A 72-year-old man with a history of constipation presents with increased temperature, diarrhoea and left iliac fossa pain. On examination there is tenderness in the left iliac fossa.

ANSWERS: see page 35

3 Small bowel obstruction

A   adhesions   F   intussusception
B   strangulated inguinal hernia   G   intra-abdominal abscess
C   small bowel atresia   H   Meckel's diverticulum
D   Crohn's disease   I   midgut volvulus
E   irritable bowel syndrome

For each clinical scenario below give the most likely cause for the clinical findings. Each option may be used only once.

1   A 54-year-old woman presents to A&E with a 48-hour history of colicky abdominal pain, vomiting and abdominal distension. Basic observations on arrival are: pulse 120/min, BP 100/75 mmHg, temperature 38°C. Abdominal examination reveals generalized tenderness, with a firm, tender, 3×4 cm swelling in the right groin. Bowel sounds are absent.

2   A 13-year-old boy underwent an appendicectomy 7 days ago for suppurative appendicitis. Over the past 48 hours he has complained of right iliac fossa pain, vomiting and abdominal distension. Bowel sounds are absent. Basic observations on arrival are: pulse 110/min, BP 105/64 mmHg, temperature 37.2°C. His mother is a nurse and says that he has had spiking temperatures of above 38°C at home.

3   A 76-year-old man with a history of hemicolectomy 3 years ago presents to his GP with worsening colicky abdominal pain associated with vomiting, and abdominal distension. Basic observations on arrival are: pulse 98/min, BP 165/75 mmHg, temperature 37.8°C. On abdominal examination there is a distended abdomen with no tenderness, rebound or guarding. Bowel sounds are tinkling.

4   A 23-year-old man with a 6-month history of weight loss, anorexia, recurrent abdominal pain after eating, and diarrhoea presents to A&E. The pain is colicky associated with vomiting, absolute constipation, and abdominal distension over the past 3 days. Basic observations on arrival are: pulse 120/min, BP 89/56 mmHg, temperature 38.2°C. He is tender in the central abdominal region without guarding or rebound. Blood tests: Hb 10.1 g/dL, WCC 18.0×10^9/L, CRP 155 mg/L, Alb 28 g/L.

ANSWERS: see page 36

4 Abdominal masses

A	renal cell carcinoma	G	diverticulosis
B	ovarian carcinoma	H	hepatocellular carcinoma
C	gastric carcinoma	I	caecal carcinoma
D	sigmoid carcinoma	J	psoas abscess
E	fibroids	K	abdominal aortic aneurysm
F	pancreatic pseudocyst	L	ovarian cyst

For each clinical scenario below give the most likely cause for the clinical findings. Each option may be used only once.

1   A 65-year-old man collapses in the street. On examination he has an abdominal mass lying above the umbilicus that is expansile and pulsatile.

2   A 75-year-old man with a 3-month history of dyspepsia presents with weight loss and abdominal distension. On examination, a 3.5 cm, hard, irregular tender epigastric mass can be felt which moves on respiration. Percussion of the distended abdomen reveals shifting dullness. The left supraclavicular node is palpable.

3   A 70-year-old woman presents with a mass in the right iliac fossa and severe microcytic anaemia. On examination the mass is firm, irregular and 4 cm in diameter. The lower edge is palpable.

4   A 35-year-old woman is worried about an abdominal mass that has grown over the last 6 months and a similar length history of very heavy menstrual bleeding with no intermenstrual bleeding. On examination, a knobbly mass can be felt in the middle lower quadrant that is dull to percussion. The lower edge is not palpable. She is otherwise well.

5   A 70-year-old alcoholic presents with a tender upper abdominal mass. CT shows a thick-walled, rounded, fluid-filled mass adjacent to the pancreas.

ANSWERS: see page 38

5 Anorectal conditions

A	fissure-in-ano	G	anal carcinoma
B	perianal warts	H	rectal prolapse
C	proctalgia fugax	I	pruritus ani
D	second-degree haemorrhoids	J	ischiorectal abscess
E	fistula-in-ano	K	third-degree haemorrhoids
F	pilonidal abscess	L	syphilitic gumma

For each clinical scenario below give the most likely cause for the clinical findings. Each option may be used only once.

1   A 28-year-old man with Crohn's disease complains of watery discharge from a puckered area 2 cm from the anal canal.

2   A 32-year-old woman who has recently given birth complains of excruciating pain on defecation that persists for hours afterwards. Rectal examination is not possible due to pain.

3   A 30-year-old taxi driver complains of tenderness from an area in the midline of the natal cleft about 4 cm above the anus. This problem has been remitting and recurring for 2 years and has started to discharge today for the first time.

4   A 27-year-old pregnant woman presents with constipation and bright red blood coating her stools. On examination, two bluish tender spongy masses are found protruding from the anus. These do not reduce spontaneously and require digital reduction.

5   A 19-year-old woman presents with multiple papilliferous lesions around the anus.

ANSWERS: see page 40

6 Management of colorectal cancer

A	right hemicolectomy	F	sigmoidectomy
B	extended left hemicolectomy	G	extended right hemicolectomy
C	Hartmann's procedure	H	abdominoperineal resection
D	anterior resection	I	total colectomy
E	subtotal colectomy		

Choose the most likely operation that is required from the options above. Each answer may be used only once.

1   A 65-year-old man is found to have a rectal carcinoma that is invading the anal sphincter.

2   A 69-year-old man is brought to A&E with an acute abdomen. He is resuscitated and then taken to theatre for explorative laparotomy. He is found to have a perforated sigmoid colon secondary to a mass with malignant features.

3   A 49-year-old man with a history of weight loss and anaemia of unknown origin is found to have a large caecal tumour on colonoscopy.

4   A 58-year-old man with a history of fresh rectal bleeding is found to have a tumour of the middle third of the rectum.

ANSWERS: see page 42

7 Management of inflammatory bowel disease

A	intravenous mesalazine	F	proctocolectomy with ileostomy
B	steroid enemas	G	elemental diet
C	stricturoplasty	H	subtotal colectomy and ileostomy
D	high-dose intravenous steroids	I	fistulectomy
E	proctocolectomy with ileal pouch	J	extensive small bowel resection

Choose the most suitable management from the options above. Each answer may be used only once.

1   A 65-year-old patient has been suffering from frequent debilitating exacerbations of ulcerative colitis and would like curative surgery.

2   A 28-year-old patient suffers from ulcerative colitis refractory to medical therapy. He agrees that surgery is required to treat his severe symptoms but does not want a stoma.

3   A 30-year-old patient with ulcerative colitis is brought to A&E suffering with severe abdominal pain. A diagnosis of toxic megacolon is made.

4   A 28-year-old patient with Crohn's disease presents with complete small bowel obstruction. Small bowel follow-through shows short small bowel strictures.

ANSWERS: see page 43

8 Investigation of gastrointestinal bleeding

A	barium swallow	F	ERCP
B	flexible sigmoidoscopy	G	oesophagogastroduodenoscopy
C	watch and wait	H	small bowel follow-through
D	faecal occult blood	I	colonoscopy
E	CT abdomen		

For each clinical scenario below give the most appropriate investigation. Each option may be used only once.

1   A 42-year-old alcoholic presents with haematemesis.

2   A 65-year-old man presents with a history of weight loss and diarrhoea. He has noticed blood mixed in with stools.

3   A 74-year-old woman presents with a 3-month history of worsening constipation and rectal bleeding.

4   A 65-year-old man with a history of diverticular disease is admitted to the surgical ward with suspected diverticulitis. He has been treated with antibiotics and intravenous fluids but is not improving after 24 hours.

ANSWERS: see page 44

9 Paediatric surgery

A	hydrocoele	F	Wilms' tumour
B	coeliac disease	G	Hirschsprung's disease
C	intussusception	H	pyloric stenosis
D	gastroschisis	I	necrotizing enterocolitis
E	duodenal atresia	J	infantile colic

For each clinical scenario below give the most likely cause for the clinical findings and appropriate management. Each option may be used only once.

1   A 7-month-old child is brought to A&E crying inconsolably and drawing his legs up. He has had one episode of vomiting and has been passing bloody stools. On examination a small mass is palpable in the right upper quadrant.

2   A 6-week-old child is brought to A&E by his mother as she has been concerned about severe forceful vomiting shortly after feeding. He is reported to be constantly hungry. There is no history of diarrhoea. On examination the child looks dehydrated and malnourished. Gastric peristalsis is visible.

3   A newborn has failed to pass meconium in the first 48 hours and is reluctant to feed. On examination the abdomen is distended. Plain abdominal radiography shows distended loops of bowel with absence of air in the rectum.

4   A newborn with trisomy 21 has suffered several episodes of bilious vomiting from a few hours since birth. On examination the baby has a scaphoid abdomen. Plain abdominal film shows a large gastric bubble proximal to an air-filled first part of duodenum.

ANSWERS: see page 44

10 Splenomegaly

A	malaria	G	spherocytosis
B	pernicious anaemia	H	infectious mononucleosis
C	sarcoidosis	I	cutaneous leishmaniasis
D	idiopathic thrombocytopenic	J	Budd–Chiari syndrome
	purpura	K	myeloma
E	Gaucher's disease	L	Felty syndrome
F	infective endocarditis	M	acute lymphoblastic leukaemia

For each clinical scenario below give the most likely cause for the clinical findings. Each option may be used only once.

1   A 75-year-old woman has noticed a fullness in the left upper quadrant. On examination, the GP feels that there is a smooth moderately enlarged spleen. There is a past medical history of rheumatoid arthritis and high blood pressure. Routine blood tests show a normocytic anaemia and low white cell count.

2   A 23-year-old man presents with a week's history of fever and sore throat. He developed a macular rash after being prescribed ampicillin by his GP. On examination he has enlarged posterior cervical nodes, palatal petechiae and splenomegaly.

3   A 21-year-old female backpacker returning from India presents with flu-like symptoms followed by a periodic fever. She is anaemic, jaundiced and has moderate splenomegaly.

4   A 28-year-old woman presents with abdominal pain, vomiting and jaundice. On examination she has tender hepatosplenomegaly and ascites. She has a history of recurrent miscarriages.

5   A 16-year-old child is being investigated for gallstones. Routine blood tests show mild anaemia and clinically there is smooth painless splenomegaly. The haematologist recommends a direct Coomb's test which is negative. Blood film shows the presence of reticulocytes and spherocytes.

ANSWERS: see page 46

11 Ulcers

A   basal cell carcinoma   G   ischaemic ulcer
B   Bowen's disease   H   neuropathic ulcer
C   squamous cell carcinoma   I   gumma
D   aphthous ulcer   J   tuberculous ulcer
E   Marjolin's ulcer   K   verruca
F   venous ulcer

Select from the options above the type of ulcer that is being described in the questions below. Each option may be used only once.

1   A 62-year-old man presents with a flat sloping-edged ulcer over the left medial malleolus.

2   A tanned 66-year-old man presents with an ulcerated lesion on the nose, with a rolled edge.

3   A 60-year-old man complains of a bleeding ulcer on the upper region of the left cheek. It has an everted edge and there are some palpable cervical lymph nodes.

4   A 71-year-old man presents with an exquisitely painful punched-out ulcer on the tip of the right big toe. On examination, the surrounding area is cold.

5   A 58-year-old diabetic presents with a painless punched-out ulcer on the sole of the right foot. The surrounding area has reduced pain sensation.

ANSWERS: see page 48

12 Abnormal abdominal x-rays

A	Crohn's disease	G	sigmoid volvulus
B	diverticulosis	H	intussusception
C	chronic pancreatitis	I	ulcerative colitis
D	acute pancreatitis	J	pyloric stenosis
E	gluten-sensitive enteropathy	K	small bowel obstruction
F	acute appendicitis	L	perforated duodenal ulcer

For each clinical scenario below give the most likely cause for the clinical findings. Each option may be used only once.

1   A 55-year-old with several months' history of epigastric discomfort presents acutely unwell in A&E. An x-ray film shows free gas under the diaphragm.

2   Abdominal film of an elderly constipated woman shows a dilated 'inverted U' loop of bowel.

3   A 31-year-old man presents with fever and bloody diarrhoea. He is tachycardic and has Hb 10.0 g/dL. Abdominal film shows loss of haustral pattern and a colonic dilatation of 8 cm.

4   A 26-year-old student presents with bloody diarrhoea, abdominal pain and weight loss. Barium enema reveals 'cobblestoning' and colonic strictures.

5   A 45-year-old man presents with severe epigastric pain and vomiting. Abdominal film shows absent psoas shadow and 'sentinel loop' of proximal jejunum.

ANSWERS: see page 49

13 Complications of gallstones

A	biliary colic	F	acute cholecystitis
B	gallbladder carcinoma	G	empyema
C	acute pancreatitis	H	chronic cholecystitis
D	gallstone ileus	I	mucocoele
E	ascending cholangitis		

Choose the most likely complication from the choices above. Each answer may be used only once.

1   A 45-year-old woman presents with fever and significant right upper quadrant pain. On examination there is marked jaundice and the nurse has reported that the patient is having rigors. Blood tests show plasma bilirubin 250 mmol/L, ALT 200 U/L, ALP 800 U/L, WCC 23×10^9/L.

2   A 55-year-old man presents with constant right upper quadrant pain associated with vomiting. He is afebrile.

3   A 63-year-old man presents with a 3-day history of worsening abdominal pain and vomiting. Abdominal x-ray reveals dilated loops of small bowel and air in the biliary tree.

4   A 52-year-old man presents with vomiting and severe epigastric pain radiating to the back. Abdominal x-ray shows a dilated proximal small bowel loop.

ANSWERS: see page 50

14 Breast conditions

A	Paget's disease	H	fibroadenoma
B	phylloides tumour	I	postpartum fat necrosis
C	mammary haemangioma	J	gynaecomastia
D	galactocoele	K	mastitis
E	chronic breast abscess	L	dermatitis herpetiformis
F	carcinoma of breast	M	duct ectasia
G	benign eczema of nipple		

For each clinical scenario below give the most likely cause for the clinical findings. Each option may be used only once.

1   A 75-year-old woman presents to her GP with a breast lump in the upper outer quadrant. On examination the lump is hard and irregular. There is axillary lymphadenopathy.

2   A 53-year-old woman presents with nipple retraction and a greeny-yellow discharge. Ultrasound shows dilated breast ducts.

3   A 21-year-old woman presents with a smooth, non-tender, highly mobile mass on the upper outer quadrant of the right breast. Fine needle aspiration shows benign breast epithelial cells (C2).

4   A 70-year-old woman presents with a worsening eczema-like rash overlying the areola and nipple. The rash does not itch. On examination a palpable mass can be felt under the rash.

5   A 26-year-old woman presents a fortnight postpartum with a painful, enlarged left breast. On examination she is pyrexial and her breast is tender and inflamed. There are no palpable masses.

ANSWERS: see page 51

15 Treatment of breast cancer

A   tamoxifen
B   cytotoxic chemotherapy
C   mastectomy and immediate
    reconstruction
D   quadrantectomy
E   immunotherapy
F   radical mastectomy

G   radical mastectomy plus
    radiotherapy
H   wide local excision, sentinel
    node biopsy plus tamoxifen
I   wide local excision, axillary node
    clearance and chemotherapy
J   no further intervention

For each clinical scenario below give the most appropriate treatment. Each option may be used only once.

1   A 92-year-old woman presents with oestrogen receptor positive stage III invasive ductal carcinoma.

2   A 35-year-old woman is diagnosed with ductal carcinoma-in-situ involving all quadrants of the breast.

3   A 60-year-old patient presents with a 2 cm invasive ductal carcinoma of the outer quadrant of the right breast. The tumour is oestrogen receptor positive.

4   A 32-year-old patient presents with a 2.5 cm invasive ductal carcinoma. She has a palpable axillary lymph node which reveals cancer cells on cytology. The tumour is oestrogen receptor negative.

ANSWERS: see page 52

16 Skin lesions

A	Marjolin's ulcer	F	basal cell carcinoma
B	Kaposi's sarcoma	G	vitiligo
C	malignant melanoma	H	squamous cell carcinoma
D	keratoacanthoma	I	fat necrosis
E	keloid	J	papilloma

Choose the most likely skin lesion that is described in the scenarios from the options above. Each option may be used only once.

1   A 77-year-old patient presents with a 1.5 cm raised lesion above the right eyebrow. On examination the lesion is pearly in appearance with rolled edges and telangiectasia on its surface.

2   A 60-year-old man presents with a 2.5 cm rapidly growing lesion situated on the right side of the nose. On examination it has an everted edge with prominent keratinization.

3   A 45-year-old woman presents with a dark, 8 mm lesion on the lateral aspect of the right lower leg. It occasionally bleeds on contact.

4   A 35-year-old woman complains of a browny-red pedunculated lesion situated along her appendicectomy scar.

ANSWERS: see page 54

17 Presentation with a lump

A	histiocytoma	H	neurofibroma
B	myosarcoma	I	sebaceous cyst
C	ganglion	J	keloid
D	abscess	K	Marjolin's ulcer
E	lipoma	L	keratoacanthoma
F	carbuncle	M	osteoma
G	furuncle		

For each description of a lump(s) below give the most likely cause for the clinical findings. Each option may be used only once.

1 A 22-year-old man presents with a lump on the scalp. Examination reveals a smooth, spherical tense lump. A small punctum can be seen on the surface.

2 A 33-year-old man presents with a swelling on the upper arm which has been growing slowly for a number of years. Examination reveals a soft, compressible, non-tender lobulated mass.

3 A 28-year-old man presents with a painless swelling on the dorsum of the right hand. Examination reveals a smooth, spherical, tense, 1.5 cm swelling. The overlying skin can be drawn over it.

4 A 29-year-old man presents with two mobile fusiform-shaped lumps on the forearm. Each swelling feels like firm rubber and causes tingling in the hand upon pressure.

5 A 65-year-old woman presents with a rapidly growing lump just below the eye. Examination reveals a 2 cm, smooth, round, skin-coloured lump with a black central core. The lump is freely mobile over subcutaneous tissues.

ANSWERS: see page 55

18 Pathology terminology

A   agenesis   F   hypoplasia
B   dysplasia   G   aplasia
C   hyperplasia   H   metaplasia
D   hypertrophy   I   neoplasia
E   atrophy

Choose the pathological term being described by the definitions below. Each option may be used only once.

1   The transformation of one fully differentiated cell type into another fully differentiated cell type.

2   An increase in the number of cells within tissue.

3   Abnormal, excessive uncoordinated growth of tissue.

4   An increase in the size of cells within tissue.

ANSWERS: see page 56

19 Thyroid conditions (i)

A   follicular carcinoma   F   Riedel's thyroiditis
B   Hashimoto's disease   G   Graves' disease
C   anaplastic carcinoma   H   follicular adenoma
D   papillary carcinoma   I   medullary carcinoma
E   lymphoma   J   De Quervain's thyroiditis

For each clinical scenario below give the most likely cause for the clinical findings. Each option may be used only once.

1   A 75-year-old woman presents with acute airway obstruction and a thyroid mass after several weeks of worsening shortness of breath. Postmortem reveals a thyroid mass that has invaded the trachea and surrounding structures. Histology shows giant cells containing pleomorphic hyperchromatic nuclei.

2   A 38-year-old patient presents with a 2.5 cm right-sided thyroid mass. On examination there is mild enlargement of the cervical lymph nodes. A thyroidectomy is performed and histology reveals a non-encapsulated infiltrative mass. Psammoma bodies and epithelial cells with large clear areas within the nuclei are noted.

3   A 24-year-old woman presents with a diffusely enlarged thyroid gland. On examination she has a fine tremor and exophthalmos.

4   A 30-year-old woman presents with a tender thyroid swelling associated with fever. Investigations reveal no evidence of infection.

ANSWERS: see page 57

20 Thyroid conditions (ii)

A   follicular carcinoma
B   Hashimoto's disease
C   anaplastic carcinoma
D   endemic goitre
E   lymphoma
F   Riedel's thyroiditis

G   Graves' disease
H   follicular adenoma
I   medullary carcinoma
J   De Quervain's thyroiditis
K   papillary carcinoma

For each clinical scenario below give the most likely cause for the clinical findings. Each option may be used only once.

1   A 36-year-old woman presents with a history of increasing weight gain, tiredness and neck swelling. On examination the patient has a firm rubbery goitre. Fine needle aspiration shows a diffuse lymphocytic and plasma cell infiltrate. The report also mentions the presence of lymphoid follicles and parenchymal atrophy.

2   A 40-year-old woman presents with a history of a slowly growing right-sided lump at the base of the neck. On examination there is a thyroid nodule with associated lymphadenopathy. She has a recent history of adrenalectomy.

3   A 45-year-old woman presents with a painless, firm, left-sided neck swelling. Fine needle aspiration reveals the presence of multiple compact follicles. Histology shows evidence of capsular and blood vessel invasion.

4   A 55-year-old African man is referred to the ENT clinic with a large, smooth goitre that has been increasing in size for at least 20 years.

ANSWERS: see page 58

21 Feeding the surgical patient

A	elemental diet	F	high-protein liquid supplements
B	normal oral intake	G	50% dextrose i.v.
C	total parenteral nutrition (TPN)	H	Hartmann's solution i.v.
D	nasojejunal feeding	I	percutaneous endoscopic
E	percutaneous endoscopic gas-		jejunostomy
	trostomy (PEG)	J	nasogastric feeding

Choose the most suitable means of providing nutrition from the options above. Each option may be used only once.

1   A 29-year-old man is admitted to the surgical ward following an acute exacerbation of Crohn's disease. He had a limited small bowel resection several months ago and has subsequently developed a high enterocutaneous fistula. On examination he appears malnourished.

2   A 40-year-old woman is involved in a road traffic accident and suffers significant head injuries with associated maxillofacial trauma. A prolonged recovery is expected.

3   A 57-year-old man with oesophageal cancer is severely malnourished due to significant dysphagia to solid food. He is able to tolerate small volumes of liquid feed with discomfort.

4   A 25-year-old homeless patient who has not eaten for 24 hours requires, later in the day, an incision and drainage procedure for a groin abscess.

ANSWERS: see page 60

22 The shocked surgical patient

A	hypovolaemia	F	left ventricular failure
B	sepsis	G	pulmonary embolism
C	cardiac tamponade	H	anaphylaxis
D	tension pneumothorax	I	acute adrenal failure
E	neurogenic shock	J	diabetic ketoacidosis

For each clinical scenario below give the most likely cause for the clinical findings. Each option may be used only once.

1   A 65-year-old patient is brought to A&E following a trauma call. On examination he has right-sided chest wall tenderness and trauma. X-rays reveal a proximal displaced femoral fracture. On examination the airway is patent, chest wall expansion is generally reduced and breath sounds vesicular bilaterally. Heart sounds are normal; jugular venous pressure is not visible; respiratory rate 20/min, pulse 110/min, BP 90/60 mmHg.

2   A 35-year-old patient complains of shortness of breath and palpitations shortly after admission to the surgical ward from A&E for management of acute cholecystitis. Observation shows a sudden drop in blood pressure to 90/40 mmHg with accompanying tachycardia. On examination there is marked erythema around the intravenous cannula on the dorsum of the left hand.

3   A 68-year-old patient is brought back to the ward following uncomplicated abdominal artery aneurysm repair. He had been suffering from significant pain postoperatively and was seen by the acute pain team about 15 minutes ago. The nurse calls you to review as the blood pressure has dropped to 90/50 mmHg. Pulse is 60/min. He feels a little dizzy but is not in pain. Urine output has been adequate postoperatively and CVP is +12.

4   A 74-year-old patient is brought to A&E after being found collapsed at home. On examination the patient has a rigid abdomen. Pulse 120/min, BP 100/60 mmHg, temperature 38°C.

ANSWERS: see page 61

23 Chest trauma

A	isolated rib fracture	G	haemothorax
B	aortic dissection	H	diaphragmatic rupture
C	simple pneumothorax	I	diaphragmatic contusions
D	flail chest	J	myocardial contusion
E	aortic dissection	K	pleural effusion
F	cardiac tamponade	L	tension pneumothorax

For each clinical scenario below give the most likely cause for the clinical findings. Each option may be used only once.

1   A 45-year-old male is brought to A&E after suffering multiple stab wounds to the chest. On examination the patient is in respiratory distress with poor expansion on the right side of the chest. There is deviation of the trachea to the left. Neck veins appear distended. SaO_2 is 90 per cent on air, pulse 120/min, BP 90/55 mmHg.

2   A 45-year-old patient is involved in a road traffic accident and is noted to have bruising all over the chest. On examination he has a shallow tachypnoea with indrawing of the chest wall on inspiration. SaO_2 is 94 per cent on air, pulse 110/min, BP 100/65 mmHg.

3   A 45-year-old man is stabbed in the right side of the chest. Chest x-ray shows a whiteout of the right lung field.

4   A 26-year-old man is brought to A&E *in extremis* after suffering a single stab wound to the left side of the chest. On examination the patient is tachypnoeic, heart sounds are muffled and blood pressure is 90/55 mmHg despite intravenous fluid resuscitation.

ANSWERS: see page 62

24 Glasgow Coma Scale

A	0	F	10
B	3	G	11
C	4	H	12
D	7	I	13
E	9	J	14

Calculate the Glasgow Coma Score (GCS) of the patients in the scenarios below.

1   An 86-year-old man is brought to A&E with a suspected subarachnoid haemorrhage. On examination he is moaning incomprehensibly with his eyes closed. Nail-bed pressure causes limb flexion and eye-opening.

2   An 8-year-old girl presents with fever, neck stiffness and photophobia. She is confused, with spontaneous eye-opening and can obey motor commands.

3   A homeless man is brought to A&E by paramedics after being discovered by a commuter in an unconscious state. There are no motor responses to pain and eye-opening and verbal responses cannot be elicited.

4   A 78-year-old woman is found unresponsive to pain or speech on the ward by a nurse 3 days after carotid endarterectomy. On examination there is no speech, no eye-opening to pain, and there is abnormal rigid extension of her arms and legs.

ANSWERS: see page 64

25 Complications of blood transfusion

A	hyperkalaemia	G	thrombophlebitis
B	iron overload	H	air embolus
C	transfusion-related acute lung injury	I	delayed haemolytic transfusion reaction
D	hypothermia	J	hypocalcaemia
E	non-haemolytic febrile reaction	K	viral infection
F	haemolytic transfusion reaction	L	circulatory overload

Choose the most likely complication from the options above. Each option may be used only once.

1   A 75-year-old patient is found to be acutely short of breath after receiving her third unit of packed red cells. On examination there are fine end inspiratory crackles up to mid zones in both lung fields.

2   A 37-year-old patient complains of headache and abdominal pain a few minutes after red cell transfusion. Temperature 38.5°C, pulse 120/min, BP 100/60 mmHg.

3   A 50-year-old patient presents with jaundice 5 days after receiving a red cell transfusion.

4   A 24-year-old patient is noted to be flushed a few minutes after starting a red cell transfusion. Temperature 37.8°C. The temperature and symptoms respond to paracetamol.

ANSWERS: see page 65

26 Head injury

A	scalp haematoma	F	subdural haematoma
B	concussion syndrome	G	post-concussive syndrome
C	diffuse axonal injury	H	cerebral contusion
D	basal skull fracture	I	extradural haemorrhage
E	subarachnoid haemorrhage		

For each clinical scenario below give the most likely cause for the clinical findings. Each option may be used only once.

1   A 24-year-old student is brought to A&E after being assaulted outside a club. On examination, GCS is 14 (confused) and he is under the influence of alcohol. CT reveals small areas of haemorrhage throughout the frontal region. He is admitted to the surgical ward for neuro-observations; 24 hours later the nurses report that he is increasingly confused and restless with a GCS of 12 (confused, localizing and eye-opening to speech).

2   A 75-year-old woman is brought to A&E by her husband who reports that her consciousness level has been fluctuating. He reports that she banged her head following a fall a few days ago but did not lose consciousness at the time. CT shows a hyperdense crescentic lesion against the inner aspect of the left frontal skull. There is moderate midline shift.

3   A 42-year-old man is found unconscious on the street. On examination there is bruising around both eyes and a clear nasal discharge.

4   A 25-year-old was involved in a high-speed road traffic accident 48 hours ago. He has been comatosed since the injury. There are no major abnormalities on CT.

ANSWERS: see page 66

27 Hepatomegaly

A	Reidel's lobe	F	infectious mononucleosis
B	Wilson's disease	G	amyloidosis
C	hydatid disease	H	lymphoma
D	malaria	I	hepatitis re-activation
E	hepatocellular carcinoma	J	Budd–Chiari syndrome

For each clinical scenario below give the most likely cause for the clinical findings. Each option may be used only once.

1   A 65-year-old man with a history of previous hepatitis B infection presents with a craggy mass in the right upper quadrant.

2   A 42-year-old farmer presents with a history of shortness of breath and abdominal pain. Clinical examination shows enlargement of the liver. Ultrasound reveals numerous cystic lesions within the liver.

3   A 26-year-old man presents with significant bilateral cervical lymphadenopathy, shortness of breath and marked hepatosplenomegaly. CT reveals extensive mediastinal, para-aortic and pelvic lymphadenopathy and confirms moderate enlargement of the liver and spleen.

4   A 31-year-old pregnant woman presents with a history of upper abdominal pain and jaundice. Examination of the abdomen reveals hepatomegaly and ascites.

ANSWERS: see page 68

28 Bleeding diatheses

A	disseminated intravascular coagulopathy	F	antithrombin III deficiency
B	hereditary spherocytosis	G	hereditary haemorrhagic telengiectasia
C	warfarin	H	protein C deficiency
D	sickle cell anaemia	I	factor VIII deficiency
E	factor V Leiden			

For each clinical scenario below give the most likely cause for the clinical findings. Each option may be used only once.

1   A 75-year-old woman with a previous history of stroke on the waiting list for laparascopic cholecystectomy is found to bruise easily.

2   A 38-year-old on the intensive care unit with sepsis following bowel surgery is found to have bleeding from the wound site. Prothrombin time (PT), and activated partial thromboplastin time (APTT) are markedly prolonged.

3   A 17-year-old woman presents with recurrent persistent epistaxes. There is a family history of the problem and her father required numerous operations to treat the nose bleeds.

4   A 9-year-old boy is referred to the orthopaedic department with a haemarthrosis of the right knee following a minor accident in the playground.

ANSWERS: see page 69

29 Congenital heart disease

A   tetralogy of Fallot
B   ventricular septal defect
C   tricuspid regurgitation
D   Marfan syndrome
E   atrial septal defect

F   patent ductus arteriosus
G   bicuspid aortic valve
H   atrial myxoma
I   coarctation of the aorta

For each clinical scenario below give the most likely cause for the clinical findings. Each option may be used only once.

1   A 55-year-old patient is referred to the cardiothoracic surgeons with episodes of chest pain and syncope. On examination there is a marked ejection systolic murmur.

2   A 3-month-old baby is referred with failure to thrive and episodes of cyanosis. On examination there is marked clubbing of the fingers and toes.

3   A 34-year-old male is found to have an early diastolic murmur. On examination he is tall and slim with hypermobile joints. His father died in his early forties.

4   A 26-year-old girl with Turner syndrome presents with raised blood pressure. On examination the femoral pulses are diminished.

ANSWERS: see page 70

30 Eponymous surgical procedures

A   Ramstedt's procedure
B   Hartmann's procedure
C   Nissen's fundoplication
D   Lord's procedure
E   Bankart repair

F   Blalock–Thomas–Taussig procedure
G   Bilroth operation
H   Whipple's procedure
I   Sistrunk's procedure

For each of the following patients choose the most appropriate procedure from the list above. Each option may be used only once.

1   A patient requiring surgery for a thyroglossal cyst.

2   A patient with a tumour in the head of the pancreas.

3   A patient with a symptomatic paraoesophageal hiatus hernia.

4   A child with severe pyloric stenosis.

ANSWERS: see page 72

31 Clinical trials

A	randomized double blind placebo controlled study	F	anecdotal report
B	case control study	G	crossover study
C	cohort study	H	expert opinion
D	cross sectional study	I	meta-analysis of randomized controlled trials
E	case series		

Choose the type of study from the options above. Each option may be used only once.

1   The study associated with the highest level of evidence.

2   Individuals with varying degrees of sunlight exposure are followed up for many years and observed for the incidence of skin cancer.

3   A notes review of 100 people treated with transoral laser therapy is used to measure the incidence of dry mouth.

4   A group of schoolboys is given a questionnaire survey to find out the number that had a history of appendicectomy.

ANSWERS: see page 73

ANSWERS

1 The acute abdomen

ANSWERS: 1K, 2B, 3F, 4C, 5D

> A 36-year-old man complains of waves of pain in the lower left flank.

K Renal colic is excruciatingly painful and usually requires opiates for adequate analgesia. It classically gives rise to waves of pain as the peristaltic contractions of the ureter attempt to expel the stone. There may be radiation of pain to the groin or inner thigh. Urine dipstick almost always shows evidence of haematuria and the absence of red blood cells in the urine makes a diagnosis of renal colic less likely. Around 60% of stones are radio-opaque and therefore a KUB film (kidney, ureters, bladder) will often identify the pathology. Non-contrast helical CT is the investigation of choice to identify kidney/ureteric stones.

> A 45-year-old man presents in A&E with severe epigastric pain radiating to the back and vomiting. On examination he is tachycardic with low blood pressure and respiratory distress. Past medical history includes gallstones and reflux oesophagitis.

B Gallstones and excessive alcohol intake are the two most common causes of acute pancreatitis. Acute pancreatitis is a medical emergency and can carry a high mortality despite early treatment. The haemodynamic instability and development of respiratory symptoms may suggest the development of SIRS (systemic inflammatory response syndrome) or ARDS (acute respiratory distress syndrome). There are several clinical scoring systems to assess the severity of acute pancreatitis e.g. Ranson criteria and APACHE II. Severity can also be assessed on CT imaging by the Balthazar scoring system.

> A 44-year-old obese woman presents with continuous right upper quadrant pain, vomiting and fever. There is marked right upper quadrant tenderness when palpating on inspiration.

F Acute cholecystitis is inflammation of the gallbladder following obstruction of the cystic duct (usually by a stone) that has given rise to infection. There are symptoms and signs of infection e.g. high temperature, increased white cell count, inflammatory markers. Murphy's sign is an indicator of acute cholecystitis. The hand is placed over the right upper quadrant and the patient is asked to breathe in. The pain resulting from the inflamed gallbladder moving downwards and striking the hand is severe and arrests the inspiratory effort. Murphy's sign is negative in simple biliary colic.

A 57-year-old man is brought to the emergency department complaining of severe generalized abdominal pain. On examination he looks systemically unwell and has a rigid abdomen. His wife reports a long history of intermittent epigastric pain after meals.

C   A rigid abdomen implies significant peritoneal inflammation and is a red flag for an acute surgical emergency. This patient has a long history of intermittent epigastric pain which may be due to a history of duodenal ulceration. There is a strong case for urgent laparotomy to investigate for a likely duodenal perforation. *Helicobacter pylori* infection and chronic non-steroidal anti-inflammatory drug (NSAID) use are important risk factors for duodenal ulceration. If the patient is *H. pylori* positive, treatment should be with appropriate antibiotics plus proton pump inhibitor therapy to reduce risk of recurrence.

A 10-year-old boy presents with fever, nausea and right iliac fossa pain.

D   Acute appendicitis classically presents as a central abdominal pain which localizes to the right iliac fossa within a few hours. On examination there may be rebound tenderness due to peritoneal inflammation. An ectopic pregnancy should always be considered with a presentation of suspected appendicitis in a woman of child bearing age. Acute appendicitis is a clinical diagnosis which may be aided with the use of ultrasound or CT when appropriate.

2 Chronic abdominal pain

ANSWERS: 1H, 2E, 3J, 4M

A 35-year-old man presents with weight loss, diarrhoea and abdominal pain. On examination he has aphthous ulcers in the mouth and a mass is palpable in the right iliac fossa. Blood tests reveal low serum B_{12} and folate.

H   Crohn's disease is a chronic transmural inflammatory gastrointestinal disease that can result in skip lesions anywhere from the mouth (aphthous ulceration) to the anus (e.g. fissuring/fistulae) but favours the terminal ileum/proximal colon. Small bowel disease can lead to malabsorption (e.g. iron, vitamin B_{12} and folate).

A 26-year-old male presents with recurrent burning pain in the upper abdomen and chest following meals. He is otherwise well.

E   Reflux oesophagitis is associated with symptoms of a burning epigastric pain that may radiate into the chest or throat. Symptoms may be provoked following heavy meals or eating spicy foods. Obese and pregnant patients are particularly at risk due to splinting of the diaphragm and increased pressure against the lower oesophageal sphincter. Hiatus hernia is also a significant risk factor for oesophagitis. It may also cause chronic cough and hoarseness of the voice due to laryngopharyngeal irritation. Treatment includes conservative measures, e.g. weight reduction, dietary modification, smoking cessation. Raising the head of the bed may also reduce the effect of acid washing against the lower oesophagus in the supine patient. Medical management includes the use of H_2 antagonists, e.g. ranitidine, or proton pump inhibitors such as omeprazole.

A 21-year-old student presents with a cramping diffuse abdominal pain associated with alternating constipation and diarrhoea. Colonoscopy and inflammatory markers are normal.

J   Irritable bowel syndrome is associated with a stressful lifestyle. Younger women (under age of 40) are more frequently affected. The patient may report pain relief after defecating/passing flatus. This is a diagnosis of exclusion.

A 72-year-old man with a history of constipation presents with increased temperature, diarrhoea and left iliac fossa pain. On examination there is tenderness in the left iliac fossa.

M   Diverticular disease is more common in the western world possibly due to the low dietary fibre intake. The sigmoid colon is most commonly affected giving rise to symptoms of constipation and rectal bleeding. Diverticula may become infected causing diverticulitis due to build-up of stagnant faecal material in a diverticulum with obstruction of the neck of the diverticulum and mucus secretion/bacterial overgrowth. Most simple cases of diverticulitis may be managed conservatively with/without antibiotics. Complications to watch out for include bleeding, abscess formation, fistulization and perforation.

3 Small bowel obstruction

ANSWERS: 1B, 2G, 3A, 4D

For EMQs, key early features pointing towards small bowel obstruction to note are symptoms of *vomiting* and a classical *colicky pain*. Distension is more pronounced in the distal small bowel and large bowel obstruction. Absolute constipation is a feature of both small and large bowel obstruction.

The causes of intestinal obstruction can be classified as mechanical or non-mechanical. *Mechanical* causes can be classified by the nature of the obstruction:

- *extraluminal*: adhesions, hernia, abscess, neoplasm, volvulus
- *intraluminal*: faecolith, intussusception, gallstone ileus, meconium
- *mural*: atresia, inflammatory bowel disease, diverticulosis, neoplasm.

The most common cause of *non-mechanical* obstruction in the postoperative patient is paralytic ileus which is believed to occur as a result of the handling of bowel intraoperatively. This should normally not persist for more than a few days. Electrolyte abnormalities (e.g. hypokalaemia) and anticholinergic medications can also give rise to ileus. The term pseudo-obstruction refers to the presentation of symptoms and signs mimicking mechanical obstruction but with no obstructing lesion. It is more common in elderly patients suffering from chronic medical conditions. Treatment is conservative.

A 54-year-old woman presents to A&E with a 48-hour history of colicky abdominal pain, vomiting and abdominal distension. Basic observations on arrival are: pulse 120/min, BP 100/75 mmHg, temperature 38°C. Abdominal examination reveals generalized tenderness, with a firm, tender, 3 × 4 cm swelling in the right groin. Bowel sounds are absent.

B   This is presentation of a strangulated hernia; i.e. there is compromise of the blood supply to the viscus requiring urgent surgery to prevent bowel ischaemia. This patient should be consented for bowel resection. An *incarcerated hernia* is the term used to describe an irreducible hernia.

A 13-year-old boy underwent an appendicectomy 7 days ago for a suppurative appendicitis. Over the past 48 hours he has complained of right iliac fossa pain, vomiting and abdominal distension. Bowel sounds are absent. Basic observations on arrival are: pulse 110/min, BP 105/64 mmHg, temperature 37.2°C. His mother is a nurse and says that he has had spiking temperatures of above 38°C at home.

G   Spiking temperatures in an EMQ hint towards abscess/collection formation. This patient is suffering from appendiceal abscess formation which will need operative intervention. The cause of the symptoms is likely to be non-mechanical obstruction secondary to a paralytic ileus.

A 76-year-old man with a history of hemicolectomy 3 years ago presents to his GP with worsening colicky abdominal pain associated with vomiting, and abdominal distension. Basic observations on arrival are: pulse 98/min, BP 165/75 mmHg, temperature 37.8°C. On abdominal examination there is a distended abdomen with no tenderness, rebound or guarding. Bowel sounds are tinkling.

A   The history of previous surgery is directing you towards a diagnosis of adhesions. Adhesions and hernias are the most common causes of mechanical small bowel obstruction. If conservative management is unsuccessful (nil by mouth, intravenous fluids and nasogastric decompression) then surgery may be required to lyse the adhesions. Unfortunately, intervention surgery itself is a risk factor for further adhesion formation.

A 23-year-old man with a 6-month history of weight loss, anorexia, recurrent abdominal pain after eating, and diarrhoea presents to A&E. The pain is colicky associated with vomiting, absolute constipation, and abdominal distension over the past 3 days. Basic observations on arrival are: pulse 120/min, BP 89/56 mmHg, temperature 38.2°C. He is tender in the central abdominal region without guarding or rebound. Blood tests: Hb 10.1 g/dL, WCC 18.0 × 10⁹/L, CRP 155 mg/mL, Alb 28 g/L.

D   This patient is presenting with small bowel obstruction that is likely to be as a result of Crohn's disease complications (e.g. strictures, fistulization). The key points to note in the scenario are the protracted history of weight loss, abdominal pain and altered bowel habit in a young patient, the presence of anaemia, and evidence of poor nutrition (anorexia and low albumin).

4 Abdominal masses

ANSWERS: 1K, 2C, 3I, 4E, 5F

A 65-year-old man collapses in the street. On examination he has an abdominal mass lying above the umbilicus that is expansile and pulsatile.

K   The presence of an expansile and pulsatile mass implies the presence of aneurysm. A true aneurysm is lined by all three layers of arterial wall, whereas a false aneurysm (caused by trauma, infection etc.) is lined only by connective tissue. The UK Small Aneurysm Trial suggested that elective surgical repair of aneurysm is indicated with an aneurysm diameter greater than 5.5 cm (*Lancet* 1998; 352:1649–55). Operative options include replacement with a prosthetic graft or endovascular stent graft repair. Mortality from aneurysm rupture without surgery is 100 per cent; and even if the patient reaches the hospital surgical unit alive, overall mortality is very high (80–95 per cent).

A 75-year-old man with a 3-month history of dyspepsia presents with weight loss and abdominal distension. On examination, a 3.5 cm, hard, irregular tender epigastric mass can be felt which moves on respiration. Percussion of the distended abdomen reveals shifting dullness. The left supraclavicular node is palpable.

C   Gastric carcinoma should always be considered in a patient of this age complaining of dyspepsia for over a month. The presence of Virchow's node (left supraclavicular node) and ascites implies disseminated disease and thus carries a poor prognosis. This finding is sometimes referred to as a positive Troisier's sign.

A 70-year-old woman presents with a mass in the right iliac fossa and severe microcytic anaemia. On examination the mass is firm, irregular and 4 cm in diameter. The lower edge is palpable.

I   The predominant symptoms/signs of carcinoma vary depending on the site of colon affected. Right-sided lesions in the caecum/ascending colon are associated with weight loss and anaemia, whereas symptoms of change in bowel habit and bleeding per rectum are more common in the sigmoid colon/rectum. The possibility of a caecal carcinoma must always be considered in a patient over 40 years old presenting with symptoms of acute appendicitis as the latter is not common in the older age group. Some surgeons would consider further imaging (e.g. CT) before surgery in these cases.

A 35-year-old woman is worried about an abdominal mass that has grown over the last 6 months and a similar length history of very heavy menstrual bleeding with no intermenstrual bleeding. On examination, a knobbly mass can be felt in the middle lower quadrant that is dull to percussion. The lower edge is not palpable. She is otherwise well.

E   Fibroids are the commonly used name for fibromyomata which are benign tumours of the smooth muscle of the uterus. The incidence of fibroids increases with age. They typically present with symptoms of increased menstrual blood loss in a middle-aged woman. Other common presentations include infertility and symptoms due to pressure on other structures, such as urinary frequency or constipation. Fibroids vary considerably in size and may grow such that they occupy a large part of the abdomen and compress other structures. A patient may also present with an acute abdomen following thrombosis of a fibroid's blood supply (red degeneration). Management depends on several factors, including the size of the fibroids, symptoms, patient's circumstances, etc. Surgical interventions include myomectomy, uterine artery embolism and open/laparoscopic hysterectomy. Fibroids are oestrogen-dependent, so gonadotrophin analogues are sometimes given to shrink fibroids prior to surgery.

A 70-year-old alcoholic presents with a tender upper abdominal mass. CT shows a thick-walled, rounded, fluid-filled mass adjacent to the pancreas.

F   Pancreatic pseudocysts are usually located in the lesser sac adjacent to the pancreas. They occur due to ductal leakage following inflammation of the pancreas (acute or chronic). Chronic pancreatitis is the most common cause of pancreatic pseudocyst. These patients may present non-specifically with abdominal discomfort, nausea, early satiety etc. Complications of pancreatic pseudocyst include infection (most common), obstruction (of common bile duct leading to jaundice) and perforation. Very rarely the pseudocyst can enlarge such that it erodes nearby vessels causing pseudoaneurysm formation which can be fatal. Fortunately most pseudocysts resolve spontaneously. CT is the investigation of choice and typically shows a round/ovoid fluid-filled cavity encapsulated by a fibrous wall. A pseudocyst does not have a true epithelial lining. Pancreatic pseudocysts can be treated by drainage if it is felt that there is a high risk of complication.

5 Anorectal conditions

ANSWERS: 1E, 2A, 3F, 4K, 5B

A 28-year-old man with Crohn's disease complains of watery discharge from a puckered area 2 cm from the anal canal.

E   Fistulae are a well-recognized complication of Crohn's disease. A full rectal examination is important to detect other causes of fistula-in-ano (e.g. rectal carcinoma). Management is initially conservative with use of antibiotics and drainage if there is abscess formation. If surgery is indicated then it is important to determine the anatomy of the fistula by means of a fistulogram/MRI as the course/extent determines the intervention. Fistula surgery is specialist surgery and there are several approaches/techniques that have been adopted. However, in simple terms a low anal fistula can usually be safely laid open over a probe. Such a procedure cannot be carried out for a high fistula because of risk of damage to the anal sphincters. In these cases the use of a cutting seton or more advanced surgery is indicated.

A 32-year-old woman who has recently given birth complains of excruciating pain on defecation that persists for hours afterwards. Rectal examination is not possible due to pain.

A   Anal fissures are exquisitely tender and therefore a rectal examination is simply not possible. The patient is often constipated as defecation is so painful. This results in a vicious cycle as the stools become harder, resulting in defecation becoming more difficult and painful. Management is initially medical with liberal use of stool softeners to break the cycle of pain. GTN/diltiazem ointment may be applied topically to relax the sphincter. Surgical procedures include lateral internal sphincterotomy and controlled sphincter dilatation.

A 30-year-old taxi driver complains of tenderness from an area in the midline of the natal cleft about 4 cm above the anus. This problem has been remitting and recurring for 2 years and has started to discharge today for the first time.

F   Pilonidal disease results from hair follicle occlusion along the natal cleft. This may manifest as abscess and sinus formation. This man is likely to have an abscess which will require incision and drainage. Good postoperative wound care is vital for a good result. Incision and drainage may be complicated with sinus formation that may itself need further surgical intervention. The patient should be warned about the risk of recurrence.

A 27-year-old pregnant woman presents with constipation and bright red blood coating her stools. On examination, two bluish tender spongy masses are found protruding from the anus. These do not reduce spontaneously and require digital reduction.

K   Spongy vascular tissue surrounds and helps close the anal canal. However, if these cushions enlarge, varices of the superior rectal veins can prolapse and bleed to form haemorrhoids/piles.

- First-degree haemorrhoids remain in the rectum.
- Second-degree haemorrhoids prolapse through the rectum on defecation but spontaneously reduce.
- Third-degree haemorrhoids can only be reduced with digital reduction.
- Fourth-degree haemorrhoids remain prolapsed.

Constipation resulting in prolonged straining is a common cause and so a high-fibre diet may be a useful preventive measure. Sclerotherapy and rubber-band ligation can be provided for symptomatic haemorrhoids in the outpatient setting. Thrombosed, strangulated piles or large symptomatic prolapsed haemorrhoids that are not amenable to other therapy may be treated with haemorrhoidectomy (e.g. Milligan–Morgan procedure or a stapling procedure).

A 19-year-old woman presents with multiple papilliferous lesions around the anus.

B   Human papillomavirus (HPV) infection is responsible for anogenital warts and is particularly associated with unprotected sexual contact. Also look out for the appearance of such lesions in the immunocompromised. HPV-related warts are referred to as *condylomata acuminata*. *Condyloma lata* are broad-based, flat-topped and necrotic papules that occur with secondary syphilis. On examination of perianal warts it is important to differentiate the two lesions. If there is any doubt, a biopsy should be performed.

6 Management of colorectal cancer

ANSWERS: 1H, 2C, 3A, 4D

A 65-year-old man is found to have a rectal carcinoma that is invading the anal sphincter.

H   Abdominoperineal resection is the operation of choice for lower rectal tumours where sphincter preservation is not possible. It involves the removal of the anus, rectum and part of the sigmoid colon, and the formation of a permanent colostomy.

A 69-year-old man is brought to A&E with an acute abdomen. He is resuscitated and then taken to theatre for explorative laparotomy. He is found to have a perforated sigmoid colon secondary to a mass with malignant features.

C   Hartmann's procedure involves excision of part of the left colon with end colostomy and closure or exteriorization of the distal remnant. The main indications are:

- *Relief of obstruction* – for example in a patient presenting with obstruction secondary to sigmoid colon carcinoma. The malignancy with appropriate margins can be excised and a colostomy formed. The Hartmann's procedure can be reversed at a later date.
- *Perforation of sigmoid colon* – the patient presents as an emergency with a perforated sigmoid diverticulum/secondary to undiagnosed malignancy. A primary anastomosis is not possible with the degree of inflammation and peritonitis.
- *Refractory sigmoid volvulus* – occasionally sigmoid volvulus fails to resolve by conservative measures/passing of flatus tube etc., and emergency surgery is required. If primary anastomosis is deemed likely to fail, then a Hartmann's procedure is performed in the first instance (it can be reversed later depending on the case).

A 49-year-old man with a history of weight loss and anaemia of unknown origin is found to have a large caecal tumour on colonoscopy.

A   A right hemicolectomy is the treatment of choice for a caecal tumour. Oncological clearance of colorectal tumours is based on knowledge of the blood supply/local lymph node drainage. The right hemi-colon receives blood supply from the ileocolic, right colic and right branch of the middle colic artery, so these branches need to be ligated and divided as close to their origin as possible.

A 58-year-old man with a history of fresh rectal bleeding is found to have a tumour of the middle third of the rectum.

D   Anterior resection is the treatment of choice for cancers of the upper, middle and lower rectum (only low rectal tumours that are not too close to or involving the sphincter complex). Total mesorectal excision involves excision of the mesentery and is believed to reduce the risk of local recurrence (although this is still under debate depending on the position of the tumour). These patients may need a defunctioning loop colostomy to reduce the risk of anastomotic breakdown.

7 Management of inflammatory bowel disease

ANSWERS: 1F, 2E, 3H, 4C

A 65-year-old patient has been suffering from frequent debilitating exacerbations of ulcerative colitis and would like curative surgery.

F   Proctocolectomy with ileostomy formation is a curative procedure that will remove all of the disease process at a single operation leaving the patient with a permanent end stoma. Recurrent disease is still possible with an ileal pouch, so this is not a curative procedure.

A 28-year-old patient suffers from ulcerative colitis refractory to medical therapy. He agrees that surgery is required to treat his severe symptoms but does not want a stoma.

E   Young patients with inflammatory bowel disease are understandably reluctant to opt for surgery that will leave them with a stoma. A proctocolectomy with ileal pouch formation is a procedure that involves removal of diseased bowel including the rectum with construction of a pouch from an ileal loop that is anastomosed to the dentate line. If successful, the procedure avoids a stoma and allows complete faecal continence.

A 30-year-old patient with ulcerative colitis is brought to A&E suffering with severe abdominal pain. A diagnosis of toxic megacolon is made.

H   The emergency procedure of choice for toxic megacolon is a subtotal colectomy with ileostomy formation. Anastomosis is not a viable option in the primary emergency procedure with acutely inflamed bowel. However, as the rectum is left intact and a mucous fistula is formed, there is scope for restorative surgery at a later point.

A 28-year-old patient with Crohn's disease presents with complete small bowel obstruction. Small bowel follow-through shows short small bowel strictures.

C   Crohn's disease may affect any part of the gastrointestinal tract from mouth to anus. In this way, curative surgery is less likely in Crohn's disease than ulcerative colitis. Principles of surgical intervention in

Crohn's disease are, therefore, to keep procedures to a minimum (conserving bowel if possible). In this patient where the strictures are short, use of stricturoplasty/balloon dilatation is a reasonable surgical option. If the strictures are long or not amenable to stricturoplasty, then a limited bowel resection can be carried out.

8 Investigation of gastrointestinal bleeding

ANSWERS: 1G, 2I, 3B, 4E

A 42-year-old alcoholic presents with haematemesis.

G   An oesophagogastroduodenoscopy (OGD) will allow visualization of the oesophagus, stomach and proximal duodenum to identify the source of bleeding. In patients with a history of excessive alcohol intake the haematemesis may be due to bleeding varices which may be banded by the endoscopist to reduce risk of future bleeding. Injection sclerotherapy can be also be used to treat bleeding varices.

A 65-year-old man presents with a history of weight loss and diarrhoea. He has noticed blood mixed in with stools.

I   Colonoscopy is the investigation of choice as the history is more suggestive of a right-sided colonic lesion that would be missed if a flexible sigmoidoscopy was performed. The advantage of endoscopy over imaging is that tissue samples may be taken for histological analysis. A CT scan of the abdomen is more useful after the lesion has been detected to stage the cancer before surgery/chemotherapy.

A 74-year-old woman presents with a 3-month history of worsening constipation and rectal bleeding.

B   This history is suggestive of a left-sided colonic carcinoma that could be visualized with flexible sigmoidoscopy.

A 65-year-old man with a history of diverticular disease is admitted to the surgical ward with suspected diverticulitis. He has been treated with antibiotics and intravenous fluids but is not improving after 24 hours.

E   A CT abdomen scan is indicated in this scenario of non-resolving diverticulitis. The scan will identify any complications of diverticulitis (e.g. fistulization, abscess formation or even perforation) which would affect the management of the patient.

9 Paediatric surgery

ANSWERS: 1C, 2H, 3G, 4E

A 7-month-old child is brought to A&E crying inconsolably and drawing his legs up. He has had one episode of vomiting and has

been passing bloody stools. On examination a small mass is palpable in the right upper quadrant.

C   Intussusception is the term applied to the telescoping/invagination of a segment of bowel into the lumen of an adjoining segment. The condition is a paediatric surgical emergency and usually occurs in children between 6 and 9 months old. Presenting symptoms and signs include severe intermittent abdominal pain (causing drawing up of the legs as in infantile colic), vomiting and the passage of the well-described 'redcurrant jelly' stools. This description results from the consistency of the stool that is composed of a mixture of blood, mucus and sloughed bowel mucosa. A sausage-shaped mass may also be palpable in the right hypochondrium.

Rehydration, correction of electrolyte abnormalities and nasogastric decompression are important initial measures. The condition may be treated with careful reduction using air or contrast enema. If this fails or there is obvious peritonitis/bowel perforation, surgery is indicated.

A 6-week-old child is brought to A&E by his mother as she has been concerned about severe forceful vomiting shortly after feeding. He is reported to be constantly hungry. There is no history of diarrhoea. On examination the child looks dehydrated and malnourished. Gastric peristalsis is visible.

H   Pyloric stenosis (infantile hypertrophic pyloric stenosis) is characterized by hypertrophy and hyperplasia of the muscular layers of the pylorus resulting in an elongated thickened pylorus and a narrow gastric antrum. The incidence is around 3 in 1000 with males affected four times more frequently than females. The condition is most common in first-born males. Causation is multifactorial with both genetic and environmental variables at play.

The condition usually presents within the first few weeks of life. The most common history is that of episodes of projectile vomiting leaving the affected child constantly hungry. On examination gastric peristalsis may be observed and there may be the classical olive-shaped mass just right of the epigastrium that is palpable after a test feed. Exam questions often allude to the biochemical picture of hypochloraemic, hypokalaemic metabolic alkalosis that results from the excessive vomiting.

The most important intervention is stabilization of the patient with rehydration and correction of electrolyte abnormalities. Once this has been achieved the condition may be corrected surgically with a Ramstedt's pyloromyotomy.

A newborn has failed to pass meconium in the first 48 hours and is reluctant to feed. On examination the abdomen is distended. Plain abdominal radiography shows distended loops of bowel with absence of air in the rectum.

G   Hirschsprung's disease results from the congenital absence of parasympathetic ganglion cells in the myenteric/submucous plexuses of the distal colon/rectum. The disease has an incidence of around 1 in 5000 and is around four times more common in males. Abdominal distension and failure to pass meconium in the first 48 hours of life are common presentations. Older children may present with chronic constipation but such delayed presentation is now rare. Definitive diagnosis is established by rectal biopsy revealing absence of ganglion cells. Management is surgical and involves excision/bypass of the affected aganglionic segment of bowel.

A newborn with trisomy 21 has suffered several episodes of bilious vomiting from a few hours since birth. On examination the baby has a scaphoid abdomen. Plain abdominal film shows a large gastric bubble proximal to an air-filled first part of duodenum.

E   Duodenal atresia (DA) commonly presents with bile-stained vomiting in the first few hours of life. The condition has an incidence of about 1 in 6000 but there is a strong association with Down syndrome (up to 30 per cent of DA patients have the trisomy 21 phenotype). The double bubble appearance on chest x-ray due to dilatation of stomach and duodenum is a characteristic finding that is frequently alluded to in exam questions.

Initial management involves fluid resuscitation and correction of electrolyte abnormalities. A nasogastric tube should be passed to allow decompression. Treatment is surgical and a duodenoduodenostomy is the procedure of choice.

10 Splenomegaly

ANSWERS: 1L, 2H, 3A, 4J, 5G

A 75-year-old woman has noticed a fullness in the left upper quadrant. On examination, the GP feels that there is a smooth, moderately enlarged spleen. There is a past medical history of rheumatoid arthritis and high blood pressure. Routine blood tests show a normocytic anaemia and low white cell count.

L   Felty syndrome is a condition characterized by splenomegaly and neutropenia in a patient with rheumatoid arthritis (RA). It is strongly associated with HLA-DR4 genotype and patients are usually very strongly rheumatoid factor positive. Management involves treating the underlying RA. If patients are not improving with medical therapy and are suffering from recurrent infections, splenectomy may be indicated.

A 23-year-old man presents with a week's history of fever and sore throat. He developed a macular rash after being prescribed ampicillin

by his GP. On examination he has enlarged posterior cervical nodes, palatal petechiae and splenomegaly.

H   Infectious mononucleosis is more commonly known as glandular fever and results from primary infection with Epstein–Barr virus (EBV). The appearance of a faint morbilliform eruption or maculopapular rash after the patient is treated with ampicillin is a characteristic sign of EBV infection. There is a T-cell proliferation with the presence of large atyp-ical cells that can be observed on the blood film. There is no antiviral therapy and the patient is simply advised to rest for uncomplicated infection. Complications are rare but include thrombocytopenia, aseptic meningitis and Guillain–Barré syndrome.

A 21-year-old female backpacker returning from India presents with flu-like symptoms followed by a periodic fever. She is anaemic, jaundiced and has moderate splenomegaly.

A   The fever of malaria is classically periodic (e.g. peaking every third day). This is caused by rupture of infected erythrocytes releasing matured merozoites and pyrogens. This classical paroxysm may not necessarily be present in early infection. Thick and thin blood smears are required for diagnosis. Resistance to the traditional quinine-based drugs is now widespread and newer drugs are in development.

A 28-year-old woman presents with abdominal pain, vomiting and jaundice. On examination she has tender hepatosplenomegaly and ascites. She has a history of recurrent miscarriages.

J   Budd–Chiari syndrome is a condition characterized by obstruction to hepatic venous outflow. It usually occurs in a patient with a hypercoag-ulative state (e.g. antiphospholipid syndrome, use of oral contraceptive pill, malignancy) but can also occur due to physical obstruction (e.g. tumour). The venous congestion can lead to enlargement of the spleen as well as the liver. The history of recurrent miscarriages suggests that there may be an underlying disorder (e.g. antiphospholipid syndrome) and this should be investigated thoroughly.

A 16-year-old child is being investigated for gallstones. Routine blood tests show mild anaemia and clinically there is smooth painless splenomegaly. The haematologist recommends a direct Coomb's test which is negative. Blood film shows the presence of reticulocytes and spherocytes.

G   Hereditary spherocytosis is a genetic defect in the red cell membrane structure. Most cases are inherited in an autosomal dominant fash-ion but the patient can also present without family history due to spontaneous mutation. Patients may present with jaundice at birth but can also remain asymptomatic for many years. Direct Coomb's test is negative in hereditary spherocytosis. This is an important test as spherocytes are also commonly found in autoimmune haemolytic anaemia. Treatment of choice is splenectomy as the spleen is the site of spherocyte removal.

11 Ulcers

ANSWERS: 1F, 2A, 3C, 4G, 5H

A 62-year-old man presents with a flat sloping-edged ulcer over the left medial malleolus.

F Venous ulcers are usually found around the lower third of the leg. It is important to remember that in a longstanding venous ulcer there may be malignant change to form a squamous cell carcinoma. This is known as a Marjolin's ulcer. Look out for signs of venous hypertension manifested by skin changes (e.g. lipodermatosclerosis, haemosiderin staining).

A tanned 66-year-old man presents with an ulcerated lesion on the nose, with a rolled edge.

A Basal cell carcinoma (also known as a rodent ulcer) is a locally invasive carcinoma that is more common on areas of sun-exposed skin. The carcinoma starts as a slow-growing nodule that may be itchy or sometimes bleeds. There is necrosis of the centre, leaving a rolled edge. Basal cell carcinoma does not metastasize and surrounding lymph nodes should not be enlarged.

A 60-year-old man complains of a bleeding ulcer on the upper region of the left cheek. It has an everted edge and there are some palpable cervical lymph nodes.

C Bleeding is more common in squamous cell carcinoma than basal cell carcinoma and, unlike with the latter, there may be enlarged lymph nodes. Squamous cell carcinoma has a characteristic everted edge.

A 71-year-old man presents with an exquisitely painful punched-out ulcer on the tip of the right big toe. On examination, the surrounding area is cold.

G Ischaemic ulcers can be excruciatingly painful to the extent that changing the overlying dressing can lead to pain lasting for several hours afterwards. Ischaemic ulcers are characteristically deeper than venous ulcers and can penetrate down to the bone. The surrounding area is cold due to ischaemia.

A 58-year-old diabetic presents with a painless punched-out ulcer on the sole of the right foot. The surrounding area has reduced pain sensation.

H Neuropathic ulcers occur due to impaired sensation resulting from neurological deficit of whatever cause. Diabetes mellitus is the most common cause of neuropathic ulcers. They are characteristically painless.

12 Abnormal abdominal x-rays

ANSWERS: 1L, 2G, 3I, 4A, 5D

A 55-year-old with several months' history of epigastric discomfort presents acutely unwell in A&E. An x-ray film shows free gas under the diaphragm.

L   Free gas under the diaphragm could result from any perforated viscus (e.g. colon) and is not specific for gastric/duodenal perforation.

Abdominal film of an elderly constipated woman shows a dilated 'inverted U' loop of bowel.

G   The sigmoid colon is the most common site of volvulus in the gastrointestinal tract. The condition involves the sigmoid colon twisting around its mesenteric axis causing obstruction. The condition tends to occur in the elderly. The condition can be treated by sigmoidoscopy and the insertion of a flatus tube per rectum to allow decompression.

A 31-year-old man presents with fever and bloody diarrhoea. He is tachycardic and has Hb 10.0 g/dL. Abdominal film shows loss of haustral pattern and a colonic dilatation of 8 cm.

I   This is toxic megacolon and a presentation of severe ulcerative colitis. It is a medical and surgical emergency and there is significant risk of perforation.

A 26-year-old student presents with bloody diarrhoea, abdominal pain and weight loss. Barium enema reveals 'cobblestoning' and colonic strictures.

A   Strictures and fistulae are typical of Crohn's disease. Ulceration and fissuring give rise to 'rose-thorn' ulcers. There is discontinuous involvement of the gastrointestinal tract with skip lesions, whereas ulcerative colitis is associated with continuous disease.

A 45-year-old man presents with severe epigastric pain and vomiting. Abdominal film shows absent psoas shadow and 'sentinel loop' of proximal jejunum.

D   The absence of the psoas shadow is due to a build-up of retroperitoneal fluid. The sentinel loop refers to a segment of gas-filled proximal jejunum. However, it is important to remember that an abdominal plain film can be completely normal in a patient presenting with acute pancreatitis.

13 Complications of gallstones

ANSWERS: 1E, 2A, 3D, 4C

A 45-year-old woman presents with fever and significant right upper quadrant pain. On examination there is marked jaundice and the nurse has reported that the patient is having rigors. Blood tests show plasma bilirubin 250 mmol/L, ALT 200 U/L, ALP 800 U/L, WCC 23×10^9/L.

E   Ascending cholangitis usually occurs secondary to bacterial contamination of an obstructed biliary system. The classical description of fever with rigors, right upper quadrant pain and jaundice is known eponymously as Charcot's triad. Urgent treatment is required with broad-spectrum antibiotics plus early decompression of the biliary system by endoscopic or radiological stenting. Surgical drainage may also be required. Early recognition of this complication is vital as delay results in steadily increasing ductal pressures with consequent spilling of infected bile into the portal triads. This can lead to liver abscesses and sepsis.

A 55-year-old man presents with constant right upper quadrant pain associated with vomiting. He is afebrile.

A   Biliary colic is a constant right upper quadrant pain (unlike renal colic) as it results from the spasm of gallbladder muscle against a stone lodged in Hartmann's pouch (at neck of gallbladder) or the cystic duct. Acute cholecystitis presents with biliary colic symptoms. The key difference is that in acute cholecystitis there is development of inflammation due to the mechanical obstruction that can result in superimposed bacterial infection. These patients will therefore show signs of inflammation/infection (pyrexia, tachycardia, increased white cell count).

A 63-year-old man presents with a 3-day history of worsening abdominal pain and vomiting. Abdominal x-ray reveals dilated loops of small bowel and air in the biliary tree.

D   Gallstone ileus is caused by a mechanical obstruction of the intestine by a gallstone. This results from the formation of a fistula between the gallbladder and the small intestine allowing the passage of the gallstone and consequent impaction. Imaging may reveal the typical findings of small bowel obstruction and air in the biliary tree.

A 52-year-old man presents with vomiting and severe epigastric pain radiating to the back. Abdominal x-ray shows a dilated proximal small bowel loop.

C   Acute pancreatitis is an extrabiliary complication of gallstones. Pancreatic duct obstruction leads to duct epithelium damage that extends into the gland and results in leakage and activation of pancreatic enzymes.

Other complications include:

- *Empyema*. Acute infection may result in the accumulation of pus within the gallbladder. It should be suspected in patients who are not improving despite appropriate antibiotic therapy. Look out for descriptions of a swinging pyrexia in questions where a diagnosis of abscess formation/empyema is being implied.
- *Mucocoele*. This is characterized by dilatation and enlargement of the gallbladder without infection, secondary to prolonged obstruction of the cystic duct. There is progressive distension over a period of time due to the accumulation of mucus secreted by the epithelial cells. The condition is usually asymptomatic. On clinical examination a visible, non-tender mass is palpable in the right upper quadrant.
- *Chronic cholecystitis*. This is usually associated with gallstones and may present with long-term dyspepsia. Chronic inflammation gives rise to fibrosis and thickening of the gallbladder wall.
- *Gallbladder carcinoma*. Development of carcinoma of the gallbladder is fortunately rare. It is most commonly found within a picture of chronic cholecystitis. Questions may allude to the 'porcelain gallbladder' which refers to extensive calcification of the gallbladder wall which is strongly associated with gallbladder cancer.

14 Breast conditions

ANSWERS: 1F, 2M, 3H, 4A, 5K

A 75-year-old woman presents to her GP with a breast lump in the upper outer quadrant. On examination the lump is hard and irregular. There is axillary lymphadenopathy.

F   A hard irregular lump is a cause for concern and warrants further investigation.

A 53-year-old woman presents with nipple retraction and a greeny-yellow discharge. Ultrasound shows dilated breast ducts.

M   Duct ectasia is a condition that usually occurs peri-/post-menopausally. It has been suggested that there is hypertrophy of the ductal epithelium which subsequently breaks down and causes obstruction (and hence stagnation of secretions). There is periductal inflammation that can lead to fibrosis and nipple retraction. It is important to rule out carcinoma especially as a mass/blood-stained discharge can also be seen in duct ectasia. A ductogram characteristically shows the presence of enlarged, dilated breast ducts.

A 21-year-old woman presents with a smooth, non-tender, highly mobile mass on the upper outer quadrant of the right breast. Fine needle aspiration (FNA) shows benign breast epithelial cells (C2).

H   Fibroadenomata are characteristically highly mobile and have the consistency of firm rubber. This has given rise to the description of a fibroadenoma as a 'breast mouse'. A fibroadenoma has the appearance of a well-defined rounded lesion on mammogram. Fibroadenomata should be excised not only to confirm the diagnosis (particularly as an early carcinoma in older women may mimic a fibroadenoma) but also because they enlarge over time.

Interpretation of FNA cytology findings: C1 inadequate; C2 normal/ benign; C3 probably benign; C4 probably malignant; C5 malignant. The results obtained should be used in conjunction with other findings from the triple assessment.

A 70-year-old woman presents with a worsening eczema-like rash overlying the areola and nipple. The rash does not itch. On examination a palpable mass can be felt under the rash.

A   This condition is caused by an intraductal carcinoma which spreads up to the skin of the nipple causing eczematous changes. There is gradual erosion and ulceration of the nipple. Fortunately as the carcinoma is superficial and presentation is early (due to eczematous changes), prognosis is good.

A 26-year-old woman presents a fortnight postpartum with a painful, enlarged left breast. On examination she is pyrexial and her breast is tender and inflamed. There are no palpable masses.

K   Inflammation of the breast postpartum can be due to obstruction of the ducts resulting in extravasation of milk into perilobular tissue. This usually occurs a few days postpartum and is self-limiting. Presentation a few weeks after delivery with a more persistent pyrexia and the presence of purulent discharge implies the presence of infective mastitis. It is important to stop direct breast-feeding of the child and send a sample of the breast milk for microscopy, culture and sensitivity. As *Staphylococcus aureus* is by far the most common infective agent, flucloxacillin treatment can be started in the meantime. The major complication of mastitis is the development of an abscess which is managed surgically by incision and drainage.

15 Treatment of breast cancer

ANSWERS: 1A, 2C, 3H, 4I

A 92-year-old woman presents with oestrogen receptor positive stage III invasive ductal carcinoma.

A   In very elderly patients with comorbid conditions who have a hormone responsive tumour, it is acceptable to treat them with tamoxifen only. Tamoxifen blocks the action of oestrogen on breast cancer cells. This is called *primary endocrine therapy*.

A 35-year-old woman is diagnosed with ductal carcinoma-in-situ involving all quadrants of the breast.

C   Mastectomy is a highly effective treatment of widespread ductal carcinoma-in-situ. It is usually combined with immediate breast reconstruction. There are several options of reconstruction available to patients, which include use of implants and different myocutaneous flap reconstructions. The most common flaps used are latissimus dorsi and TRAM (transversus rectus abdominis muscle) flap reconstructions. The latter can be done as a free or pedicled flap.

A 60-year-old patient presents with a 2 cm invasive ductal carcinoma of the outer quadrant of the right breast. The tumour is oestrogen receptor positive.

H   In breast cancer management, there is a tendency towards breast-conserving surgery. This is usually in the form of wide local excision or quadrantectomy. All patients who undergo this type of surgery must receive breast radiotherapy afterwards to minimize the risk of tumour recurrence.

Sentinel lymph node biopsy is one of the advances in minimally invasive staging of breast cancer. The sentinel node is the lymph node which is in direct communication with the primary breast tumour and receives lymph fluid from it. The histological status of the sentinel node is an accurate predictor of the status of the rest of the axillary lymph nodes in breast cancer patients. Identification of the sentinel node involves injecting radioactive colloid at the site of the primary tumour followed by a nuclear medicine scan under a gamma camera. At operation, combination of a blue dye and use of a gamma detection probe lead the surgeon to this lymph node. There is a very low morbidity associated with this procedure and over 60 per cent of patients in the UK çan be spared from the side-effects of axillary lymph node dissection which is the procedure of choice in patients with proven axillary disease.

A 32-year-old patient presents with a 2.5 cm invasive ductal carcinoma. She has a palpable axillary lymph node which reveals cancer cells on cytology. The tumour is oestrogen receptor negative.

I   This woman has proven axillary lymph node disease and therefore axillary lymph node dissection is warranted. The tumour is oestrogen receptor negative and therefore tamoxifen is not indicated. For a young patient with advanced disease, adjuvant chemotherapy is indicated to reduce the risk of recurrence.

Primary drug treatment in a form of endocrine or chemotherapy can be used in other circumstances too. In patients who have inoperable locally advanced tumour, primary drug therapy aims to make it possible to perform the procedure. Additionally, in patients with large primary tumours, it could shrink the tumour down so that breast-conserving therapy can be offered to the patient.

16 Skin lesions

ANSWERS: 1F, 2H, 3C, 4E

A 77-year-old patient presents with a 1.5 cm raised lesion above the right eyebrow. On examination the lesion is pearly in appearance with rolled edges and telangiectasia on its surface.

F   Basal cell carcinoma typically occurs over areas of sun-exposed skin, especially the head and neck. It is slow-growing and rarely metastasizes. However, if left to progress it can cause significant local ulceration. The common nodular basal cell carcinoma is typically described as having a translucent/pearly appearance with surface telangiectasia. It is often described as having a 'rolled' edge. Surgical excision with an appropriate margin is the standard treatment, but curettage, cryotherapy and laser ablation therapy are other treatments that are offered for particularly small lesions.

A 60-year-old man presents with a 2.5 cm rapidly growing lesion situated on the right side of the nose. On examination it has an everted edge with prominent keratinization.

H   Invasive squamous cell carcinoma (SCC) of the skin most commonly arises from malignant change of solar/actinic keratoses. This lesion typically presents as an enlarging pink keratinized plaque which is often described as having an everted edge. SCC may metastasize and so examination of regional lymph nodes is particularly relevant during examination.

Marjolin's ulcer refers to SCC arising in a chronic site of inflammation (e.g. osteomyelitic sinus). *Bowen's disease* refers to an in-situ SCC which presents as flat, red scaly patches on sun-exposed areas. In-situ carcinoma may persist or develop into invasive disease.

Histological features of SCC include pleomorphism, dermal invasion by atypical epidermal cells, intraepithelial keratinization and intracellular bridges (at high magnification).

A 45-year-old woman presents with a dark, 8 mm lesion on the lateral aspect of the right lower leg. It occasionally bleeds on contact.

C   The incidence of melanoma is rising and exposure to sunlight is the major aetiological factor. The majority of melanomas arise from pre-existing moles and any changes in size, shape or colour, bleeding or itching should prompt the doctor to perform a biopsy. Excision biopsy is the accepted method. There are different types of melanomas, including superficial spreading, nodular, lentigo maligna, acral lentiginous and amelanotic melanoma. The superficial spreading melanoma is the commonest type comprising 70 per cent of melanomas.

Tumour thickness described by Breslow (Breslow thickness) and expressed in millimetres is the most reliable independent prognostic indicator. Presence or absence of disease within the sentinel lymph node (see answer to Q3 for EMQ 15) is regarded as another very important prognostic indicator. Presence or absence of ulceration is another important prognostic indicator, as is melanoma site. For example, melanomas in head and neck and acral regions have poorer prognosis.

Surgery in the form of wide local excision is the standard management. The thickness of the primary melanoma determines the extent of surgery and the excision margins. In melanomas less than 1 mm, a 1 cm excision margin is acceptable. Between 1 and 2 mm a 2 cm excision margin is appropriate; for melanomas over 2 mm, a 3 cm excision margin is the common practice.

Intermediate thickness melanoma patients (Breslow thickness 1–4 mm) are offered sentinel node biopsy for nodal staging.

A 35-year-old woman complains of a browny-red pedunculated lesion situated along her appendicectomy scar.

E   Keloid refers to the formation of excessive scar tissue following trauma to the skin. This is believed to be due to an abnormality in the normal wound healing process involving excessive collagen accumulation. It is important to note that keloid may spread away from the initial site of trauma.

Keloid is more common in black patients, and the risk of developing scarring diminishes with age.

Treatment options for keloid are generally unsatisfactory. Examples include corticosteroid injections, excision surgery and cryotherapy. Prevention is the key management strategy. Minimizing incision size and appropriate closure of wounds with minimal tension along relaxed skin tension lines is crucial if surgery is carried out on high-risk individuals.

17 Presentation with a lump

ANSWERS: 1I, 2E, 3C, 4H, 5L

A 22-year-old man presents with a lump on the scalp. Examination reveals a smooth, spherical tense lump. A small punctum can be seen on the surface.

I   Sebaceous cysts are benign cystic lesions that most commonly occur on the scalp, face, neck, chest and back. There are no sebaceous glands on the palms of the hand and the soles of the feet. The punctum visible on the surface of the lump is virtually diagnostic of sebaceous cyst. The skin cannot be drawn over a sebaceous cyst. If punctured, the cyst may discharge keratinized material that is often described as 'toothpaste-like' in consistency. Sebaceous cysts may be excised under local anaesthetic.

A 33-year-old man presents with a swelling on the upper arm which has been growing slowly for a number of years. Examination reveals a soft, compressible, non-tender lobulated mass.

E   This is a typical history of a benign lipoma with slow growth over a number of years. They are generally non-tender and lobulation is the key diagnostic feature.

A 28-year-old man presents with a painless swelling on the dorsum of the right hand. Examination reveals a smooth, spherical, tense, 1.5 cm swelling. The overlying skin can be drawn over it.

C   A ganglion is a cystic degeneration of fibrous tissue and is usually found around joints, especially the dorsal surface of the wrist joint. Treatment is by excision under general anaesthetic. The patient should be warned about the possibility of recurrence.

A 29-year-old man presents with two mobile fusiform-shaped lumps on the forearm. Each swelling feels like firm rubber and causes tingling in the hand upon pressure.

H   Neurofibromata are often multiple and can appear at any age but usually present in adult life. The forearm is frequently affected. The presence of multiple neurofibromata may indicate the presence of neurofibromatosis (look out for café-au-lait spots, Lisch nodules in eye, acoustic neuroma etc.). These patients need to be followed up as there is a risk of sarcomatous change.

A 65-year-old woman presents with a rapidly growing lump just below the eye. Examination reveals a 2 cm, smooth, round, skin-coloured lump with a black central core. The lump is freely mobile over subcutaneous tissues.

L   Keratoacanthoma (also known as molluscum sebaceum) is a benign epidermal tumour that is often mistaken for squamous cell carcinoma. (Squamous cell carcinoma does not have the central necrotic core.) A keratoacanthoma should always be mobile over subcutaneous tissues. Excision is usually deemed to leave less scarring than allowing spontaneous remission.

18 Pathology terminology

ANSWERS: 1H, 2C, 3I, 4D

The transformation of one fully differentiated cell type into another fully differentiated cell type.

H   Metaplasia is defined as the transformation of one fully differenti-
      ated cell type into another fully differentiated cell type. It can be
      broadly classified into *epithelial metaplasia and connective metaplasia*.
      Squamous metaplasia is the most common form of epithelial metaplasia
      (e.g. ciliated respiratory epithelium in response to smoking). Glandular
      metaplasia is a less common form of epithelial metaplasia but is best
      exemplified by the condition known as Barrett's oesophagus. This refers
      to the metaplastic change from squamous oesophageal epithelium to
      columnar glandular epithelium due to acid reflux.

      An increase in the number of cells within tissue.

C   Hyperplasia and hypertrophy are often confused. Hyperplasia is an
      increase in the number of cells and can be either *physiological* or
      pathological. Physiological hyperplasia is seen in pregnancy in the
      breast, thyroid and pituitary gland secondary to hormonal influ-
      ences. Pathological hyperplasia can be seen in conditions associated
      with excessive secretion of hormones, such as Graves' disease (thyroid
      hyperplasia).

      Abnormal, excessive uncoordinated growth of tissue.

I   Neoplasia is characterized by abnormal excessive uncoordinated
      growth that persists despite the removal of any predisposing stimulus.
      Dysplasia is non-neoplastic proliferation that has the capacity to pro-
      gress to neoplasia. Clinically significant sites of dysplasia include the
      bronchus, cervix and oesophagus. Environmental factors (e.g. smok-
      ing and alcohol ingestion) may predispose to dysplasia in some sites.

      An increase in the size of cells within tissue.

D   Hypertrophy is an increase in the size of tissue due to an increase in
      the size of the cells. It may be *physiological* or *pathological*. Examples
      of physiological hypertrophy include the enlargement of the uterus
      in pregnancy and the hypertrophy of skeletal muscle with exercise.
      Examples of pathological hypertrophy are the development of cardio-
      myopathy and some congenital muscular dystrophies.

19 Thyroid conditions (i)

ANSWERS: 1C, 2D, 3G, 4J

      **A 75-year-old woman presents with acute airway obstruction and a
      thyroid mass after several weeks of worsening shortness of breath.
      Postmortem reveals a thyroid mass that has invaded the trachea and
      surrounding structures. Histology shows giant cells containing pleo-
      morphic hyperchromatic nuclei.**

C   Anaplastic carcinoma of the thyroid is an aggressive tumour which usu-
      ally affects more elderly patients. In EMQs, look out for the description

of a rapidly invasive thyroid tumour. It may arise from a pre-existing papillary/follicular carcinoma and is also closely associated with endemic goitre. Treatment involves surgical debulking of tumour and is usually a palliative procedure due to the aggressiveness of the tumour.

A 38-year-old patient presents with a 2.5 cm right-sided thyroid mass. On examination there is mild enlargement of the cervical lymph nodes. A thyroidectomy is performed and histology reveals a non-encapsulated infiltrative mass. Psammoma bodies and epithelial cells with large clear areas within the nuclei are noted.

D   Papillary carcinoma accounts for 60–70 per cent of all malignant thyroid neoplasms. It is a well-differentiated and minimally invasive tumour that carries a good prognosis even with lymphatic spread (which is common). The classical histological findings are Orphan Annie nuclei and psammoma bodies. Orphan Annie nuclei (named after a New York cartoon strip character) have characteristic clear areas within the nucleus giving them the appearance of 'orphan eyes'. Psammoma bodies are spiral rings of calcification that are a highly specific finding to papillary carcinoma.

Treatment involves subtotal or total thyroidectomy depending on the size and position of tumour. Patients should receive postoperative radio-iodine therapy to treat residual tumour and metastases.

A 24-year-old woman presents with a diffusely enlarged thyroid gland. On examination she has a fine tremor and exophthalmos.

G   Graves' disease is an autoimmune disease of the thyroid caused by the presence of auto-antibodies to the TSH receptor. Symptoms of thyrotoxicosis and ophthalmic involvement are the hallmark of Graves' disease. Eye signs include lid retraction, lid lag and exophthalmos.

A 30-year-old woman presents with a tender thyroid swelling associated with fever. Investigations reveal no evidence of infection.

J   De Quervain's thyroiditis is a usually self-limiting transient inflammation of the thyroid gland. It is more common in middle-aged women. The aetiology is unclear but post-viral inflammation has been implicated. Flu-like symptoms, local pain and tenderness may be present. There may also be derangement of thyroid function, classically with hyperthyroid followed by hypothyroid stages.

20 Thyroid conditions (ii)

ANSWERS: 1B, 2I, 3A, 4D

A 36-year-old woman presents with a history of increasing weight gain, tiredness and neck swelling. On examination the patient has a firm rubbery goitre. Fine needle aspiration shows a diffuse lymphocytic and plasma cell infiltrate. The report also mentions the presence of lymphoid follicles and parenchymal atrophy.

B   Hashimoto's disease is characterized by autoimmune destruction of the thyroid gland. It is the most common cause of primary hypothyroidism in areas of adequate iodine intake. The condition is associated with the presence of anti-thyroglobulin and anti-thyroid peroxidase antibodies but these may be absent in around 15 per cent of cases.

The patient usually presents with symptoms of hypothyroidism with or without neck swelling. The characteristic histological features include a diffuse lymphocytic and plasma cell infiltration with formation of lymphoid follicles and thyroid parenchymal atrophy. The treatment of choice is thyroid hormone replacement.

A 40-year-old woman presents with a history of a slowly growing right-sided lump at the base of the neck. On examination there is a thyroid nodule with associated lymphadenopathy. She has a recent history of adrenalectomy.

I   Medullary carcinoma of the thyroid originates in the parafollicular calcitonin producing C-cells of the thyroid gland. It usually presents as an isolated neck lump, and associated lymphadenopathy is common. Isolated medullary carcinoma usually presents later in life, but when associated with multiple endocrine neoplasia (MEN 2A/2B) it can present much earlier. This patient has a history of adrenalectomy which may have been performed to remove a phaeochromocytoma (part of MEN type 2). Calcitonin levels are sometimes used to assess evidence of residual disease after surgery and recurrent disease.

A 45-year-old woman presents with a painless, firm, left-sided neck swelling. Fine needle aspiration reveals the presence of multiple compact follicles. Histology shows evidence of capsular and blood vessel invasion.

A   Follicular carcinoma is several times more common in women than men. It is a well-differentiated encapsulated tumour that is characterized by haematogenous spread (lung, bone and brain). Fine needle aspiration cannot differentiate between follicular adenoma and carcinoma. The lesion may be removed and a frozen section examined perioperatively to discern whether the lesion is malignant. If the histology shows follicular carcinoma, more extensive thyroid resection is required (hemithyroidectomy, or subtotal or total thyroidectomy). Radio-iodine is required postoperatively to destroy residual disease and metastases.

A 55-year-old African man is referred to the ENT clinic with a large, smooth goitre that has been increasing in size for at least 20 years.

D   Endemic goitre is rare in the UK due to adequate iodine intake, but worldwide it is the most common cause of goitre. Iodine deficiency results in a relative lack of T3 and T4. This in turn triggers an increase in TSH levels (negative feedback) which is responsible for thyroid epithelium hyperplasia.

21 Feeding the surgical patient

ANSWERS: 1C, 2E, 3J, 4H

Adequate nutrition is a vital part of the overall management of surgical patients. There are two broad types of nutritional support: *enteral* (via gut) or *parenteral* (intravenous). Nutrition should be provided enterally if at all possible, because absence of nutrition via the gut is associated with atrophy and increased risk of bacterial translocation across the gut wall.

> **A 29-year-old man is admitted to the surgical ward following an acute exacerbation of Crohn's disease. He had a limited small bowel resection several months ago and has subsequently developed a high enterocutaneous fistula. On examination he appears malnourished.**

C   This patient has an enterocutaneous fistula and markedly inflamed bowel secondary to Crohn's disease. Nutrition provided enterally is not indicated as there will be insufficient absorption and enteral feeds will aggravate the inflammation. A high/proximal enterocutaneous fistula is a clear indication for TPN.

> **A 40-year-old woman is involved in a road traffic accident and suffers significant head injuries with associated maxillofacial trauma. A prolonged recovery is expected.**

E   As the patient has maxillofacial trauma it is not safe/viable to pass a nasogastric/nasojejunal tube. There is nothing to suggest that she has any abnormality in gut function and therefore enteral feeding should be attempted. As a prolonged period of recovery is expected, PEG feeding is a reasonable route of nutrition.

> **A 57-year-old man with oesophageal cancer is severely malnourished due to significant dysphagia to solid food. He is able to tolerate small volumes of liquid feed with discomfort.**

J   This patient is severely malnourished and will benefit from preoperative enteral feeding. The obstruction is in the oesophagus; so if one can bypass the obstruction with a nasogastric tube and feeding is tolerated, this is the optimal route. Although he is tolerating oral fluids, he is finding this uncomfortable and large volumes of liquid nutritional supplementation are neither viable nor effective in a severely malnourished patient.

> **A 25-year-old homeless patient who has not eaten for 24 hours requires, later in the day, an incision and drainage procedure for a groin abscess.**

H   This patient will be undergoing minor surgery and there is no indica-
         tion for preoperative feeding. She may be kept nil by mouth and given
         intravenous fluids to keep her well hydrated. In general, some form
         of nutritional support should be considered in patients if there is an
         inability to sustain an adequate dietary intake for more than 3 days.

22 The shocked surgical patient

ANSWERS: 1A, 2H, 3E, 4B

Shock may be defined as an inadequate tissue perfusion resulting from acute
circulatory compromise.

> A 65-year-old patient is brought to A&E following a trauma call. On
> examination he has right-sided chest wall tenderness and trauma.
> X-rays reveal a proximal displaced femoral fracture. On examination
> the airway is patent, chest wall expansion is generally reduced and
> breath sounds vesicular bilaterally. Heart sounds are normal; jugular
> venous pressure is not visible; respiratory rate 20/min, pulse 110/
> min, BP 90/60 mmHg.

A   Trauma victims may have numerous causes for their 'shocked' condition.
         This patient has suffered blunt chest trauma and a displaced long-bone
         fracture. Equal breath sounds make a tension pneumothorax unlikely.
         Tension pneumothorax is also associated with an increased JVP due to
         central venous compression. Cardiac tamponade is also possible but one
         might expect abnormality in the heart sounds (e.g. muffling) or a rise
         in the JVP. The most likely cause for the circulatory compromise in this
         patient is hypovolaemia secondary to blood loss from the femoral fracture.

         Femoral and pelvic fractures can be associated with significant blood
         loss (can be around 1–1.5 L). In this situation rapid intravenous fluid
         boluses are the immediate measure required to stabilize the patient's
         circulation and thus maintain tissue perfusion.

> A 35-year-old patient complains of shortness of breath and palpi-
> tations shortly after admission to the surgical ward from A&E for
> management of acute cholecystitis. Observation shows a sudden drop
> in blood pressure to 90/40 mmHg with accompanying tachycardia.
> On examination there is marked erythema around the intravenous
> cannula on the dorsum of the left hand.

H   This patient has suddenly become tachycardic and hypotensive and is
         short of breath. The key point in the examination is the presence of
         erythema around the cannula. The patient has only just been admit-
         ted for acute cholecystitis and it is unlikely to be infected. The patient
         could have suffered a pulmonary embolus but is not suffering from
         any chest pain and there is nothing in the history to suggest any

predisposing risk. The acute cholecystitis could result in systemic sepsis, but one might expect other markers to be mentioned (e.g. temperature). It is more likely that the patient is suffering from an anaphylactic reaction to the intravenous antibiotics given after arriving on the ward. Management includes high-flow oxygen, steroids, adrenaline (epinephrine) and fluid resuscitation.

A 68-year-old patient is brought back to the ward following uncomplicated abdominal artery aneurysm repair. He had been suffering from significant pain postoperatively and was seen by the acute pain team about 15 minutes ago. The nurse calls you to review as the blood pressure has dropped to 90/50 mmHg. Pulse is 60/min. He feels a little dizzy but is not in pain. Urine output has been adequate postoperatively and CVP is +12 mmHg.

E This patient has dropped his blood pressure but is maintaining a pulse on the lower side of normal. He has a CVP of +12 and, although central venous pressures should be interpreted as a trend (e.g. by looking at responses to a fluid challenge), he is unlikely to be hypovolaemic. With acute blood loss one would also expect the patient to mount a tachycardia before dropping blood pressure. Urine output is also good. The key information is that the patient has just been seen by the acute pain team. After such major surgery it is likely that the patient has had an epidural for analgesia. Given that there is a drop in blood pressure in a well-filled patient with a normal pulse/bradycardia, it is possible that an epidural bolus has been delivered for pain relief which caused a transient sympathetic block. This vasodilates the circulation and gives a rapid drop in venous pressure and, therefore, preload and cardiac output.

A 74-year-old patient is brought to A&E after being found collapsed at home. On examination the patient has a rigid abdomen. Pulse 120/min, BP 100/60 mmHg, temperature 38°C.

B This patient is pyrexial, tachycardic and hypotensive with a rigid abdomen. It is therefore most likely that he is suffering from septic shock secondary to peritonitis.

23 Chest trauma

ANSWERS: 1L, 2D, 3G, 4F

A 45-year-old male is brought to A&E after suffering multiple stab wounds to the chest. On examination the patient is in respiratory distress with poor expansion on the right side of the chest. There is deviation of the trachea to the left. Neck veins appear distended. SaO_2 is 90 per cent on air, pulse 120/min, BP 90/55 mmHg.

L Tension pneumothorax is a life-threatening medical emergency and should be treated on clinical suspicion. There is an old adage that you should not see a chest x-ray of a tension pneumothorax as treatment should not be delayed to obtain confirmatory imaging. Essentially the penetrating trauma produces a one-way valve whereby air enters the pleural space with each inspiration but cannot leave and causes collapse of the ipsilateral lung.

Clinical signs include diminished/absent breath sounds and hyper-resonance to percussion on the side of the tension pneumothorax with mediastinal shift to the contralateral side. There is mechanical compression of the superior/inferior vena cava giving rise to distended neck veins and hypotension.

Treatment involves immediate decompression with a large-bore cannula inserted into the second intercostal space on the midclavicular line on the side of tension pneumothorax before a definitive chest drain is provided.

A 45-year-old patient is involved in a road traffic accident and is noted to have bruising all over the chest. On examination he has a shallow tachypnoea with indrawing of the chest wall on inspiration. SaO$_2$ is 94 per cent on air, pulse 110/min, BP 100/65 mmHg.

D   The hallmark of flail chest is paradoxical chest movements (i.e. indrawing of the chest wall with inspiration and outward movement with expiration). This occurs when a section of the rib cage becomes independent of the rest of the chest wall (at least two ribs are fractured in at least two places). The condition is associated with significant ventilatory compromise due to severe pain as well as the obvious disruption to the mechanics of the chest wall.

Treatment involves oxygen therapy, adequate analgesia (may need thoracic epidural) and careful monitoring. The patient may need assistance with ventilation due to hypoxia (from pulmonary contusions) or inadequate spontaneous ventilation.

A 45-year-old man is stabbed in the right side of the chest. Chest x-ray shows a whiteout of the right lung field.

G   The chest x-ray findings are consistent with significant haemothorax. With a large haemothorax there will be dullness to percussion and reduced air entry on the affected side. Primary management involves insertion of a large-bore chest drain.

A 26-year-old man is brought to A&E *in extremis* after suffering a single stab wound to the left side of the chest. On examination the patient is tachypnoeic, heart sounds are muffled and blood pressure is 90/55 mmHg despite intravenous fluid resuscitation.

F   Penetrating trauma to the pericardium results in the filling of the pericardial space with blood which limits the expansion of the heart. Acute cardiac tamponade is classically associated with Beck's triad of muffled heart sounds, hypotension and raised JVP. A paradoxical rise in the

JVP on inspiration is difficult to detect clinically, but distended neck veins are easier to spot. The emergency treatment of choice is pericardiocentesis.

24 Glasgow Coma Scale

ANSWERS: 1D, 2J, 3B, 4C

The Glasgow Coma Scale was designed to assess and monitor the consciousness of patients. It is based on observing motor responsiveness, verbal performance and eye-opening to appropriate stimuli. *The lowest score attainable is 3 and the maximum score is 15.* As a rule of thumb, the *degree of brain injury* can be summarized as: severe injury 3–8; moderate injury 9–12; mild injury 13–15.

Eye-opening (E)

4	Opens eyes spontaneously.
3	Opens eyes in response to speech.
2	Opens eyes in response to pain.
1	There is no eye-opening.

Verbal response (V)

5	Oriented responses.
4	Confused – patient is able to understand questions but in a confused manner.
3	Inappropriate – words are spoken but patient is unable to make conversational exchange.
2	Incomprehensible – moaning, able to make sounds but no words.
1	No verbal response.

Motor (M)

6	Normal – obeys simple commands.
5	Localizing – a localizing response is a purposeful movement towards a changing painful stimulus. Pain stimuli include application of nail-bed pressure, supraorbital pressure and sternal rubbing.
4	Withdrawing – withdrawal of limb in response to pain.
3	Flexor – pain stimulus causes abnormal flexure of limbs (*decorticate posture*). The classical decorticate posture involves flexed arms, clenched fists and extended legs. The arms are pointed towards the body with the wrists and fingers bent and held on the chest.
2	Extensor – pain stimulus causes limb extension (*decerebrate posture*). The classical decerebrate posture involves rigid

extension of the arms and legs, downward pointing of the toes, and backward arching of the head.

1   No response to pain.

An 86-year-old man is brought to A&E with a suspected subarachnoid haemorrhage. On examination he is moaning incomprehensibly with his eyes closed. Nail-bed pressure causes limb flexion and eye-opening.

D   This patient has closed eyes which open with a painful stimulus (E2), moans incomprehensibly (V2) and flexes limbs with pain (M3). Total GCS is 7.

An 8-year-old girl presents with fever, neck stiffness and photophobia. She is confused, with spontaneous eye-opening and can obey motor commands.

J   Confusion is a sensitive marker of altered conscious state and this patient will score 4 out of 5 for verbal response. Overall GCS is 14.

A homeless man is brought to A&E by paramedics after being discovered by a commuter in an unconscious state. There are no motor responses to pain and eye-opening and verbal responses cannot be elicited.

B   This patient is likely to have a very poor prognosis with a GCS score of 3 (E1, V1, M1). Note that 3 is the lowest GCS score possible when all modalities can be assessed.

A 78-year-old woman is found unresponsive to pain or speech on the ward by a nurse 3 days after carotid endarterectomy. On examination there is no speech, no eye-opening to pain, and there is abnormal rigid extension of her arms and legs.

C   This patient may have suffered an embolic cerebrovascular accident as a complication of carotid artery surgery. The GCS is E1, V1, M2 (patient extending to pain), so the total is 4.

25 Complications of blood transfusion

ANSWERS: 1L, 2F, 3I, 4E

A 75-year-old patient is found to be acutely short of breath after receiving her third unit of packed red cells. On examination there are fine end inspiratory crackles up to mid zones in both lung fields.

L   Care should be taken when transfusing large volumes of red cells especially in the elderly. It is often prudent to transfuse slowly and to use small doses of diuretic (e.g. furosemide) between units. On examination, look out for the signs of acute pulmonary oedema secondary to fluid overload (e.g. shortness of breath with raised JVP, and fine end inspiratory crepitations bilaterally).

A 37-year-old patient complains of headache and abdominal pain a few minutes after red cell transfusion. Temperature 38.5°C, pulse 120/min, BP 100/60 mmHg.

F   This is a presentation of acute haemolytic transfusion reaction due to ABO incompatibility. This is a medical emergency as there is massive intravascular haemolysis of the transfused cells and activation of the coagulation cascade and disseminated intravascular coagulation may occur.

As soon as an incompatibility reaction is suspected the transfusion should be stopped and resuscitation of the patient instituted. Repeat grouping should be carried out on the donor and patient to confirm the diagnosis. A direct antiglobulin test (Coombs' test) should be carried out on the recipient post-transfusion sample.

A 50-year-old patient presents with jaundice 5 days after receiving a red cell transfusion.

I   A delayed haemolytic reaction also occurs when a patient develops an antibody directed against an antigen on transfused red cells. These antibodies are below detectable titres at the time of cross-matching and unable to cause lysis at the time of transfusion. Symptoms and signs include fever, anaemia, jaundice and haemoglobinuria. The diagnosis can be confirmed with a direct antiglobulin test.

A 24-year-old patient is noted to be flushed a few minutes after starting a red cell transfusion. Temperature 37.8°C. The temperature and symptoms respond to paracetamol.

E   Non-haemolytic febrile transfusion reactions are now less common due to the use of leucocyte-depleted blood. Febrile reactions are usually attributed to reactions between recipient antibodies reacting with white cell antigens/fragments in the donor blood or pyretic cytokines (e.g. IL-1) which accumulate in the blood product during storage. They are more common in patients who have had previous transfusions. As fever can be the presenting sign of more serious haemolytic reaction, it is important to closely monitor the patient's observations to ensure that there is a benign cause for the increased temperature.

26 Head injury

ANSWERS: 1H, 2F, 3D, 4C

A 24-year-old student is brought to A&E after being assaulted outside a club. On examination, GCS is 14 (confused) and he is under the influence of alcohol. CT reveals small areas of haemorrhage throughout the frontal region. He is admitted to the surgical ward for neuro-observations; 24 hours later the nurses report that he is increasingly confused and restless with a GCS of 12 (confused, local-izing and eye-opening to speech).

H   A cerebral contusion is essentially a bruise of the brain tissue. Contusions most commonly occur along the undersurface and poles of the frontal and temporal lobes. These brain areas are more susceptible to trauma against the ridges of the skull. Significant cerebral oedema may develop around these contusions that can increase intracranial pressure. For this reason, patients need to be closely monitored and may need repeat imaging. Significant contusions may require operative intervention.

A 75-year-old woman is brought to A&E by her husband who reports that her consciousness level has been fluctuating. He reports that she banged her head following a fall a few days ago but did not lose consciousness at the time. CT shows a hyperdense crescen-tic lesion against the inner aspect of the left frontal skull. There is moderate midline shift.

F   Following head injury, there may be tearing of the bridging veins between the cerebral cortex and venous sinuses giving rise to bleeding in the subdural space. A significant haematoma can give rise to increas-ing intracranial pressure, midline shift and ultimately tentorial hernation.

It is important to remember that even minor head injury can precipitate a subdural haemorrhage, especially in the elderly and alcoholics where there is more brain atrophy. Acute haemorrhage gives rise to a hyper-dense (white) crescentic lesion concave against the skull. Operative intervention involves craniotomy and evacuation of haematoma.

A 42-year-old man is found unconscious on the street. On examina-tion there is bruising around both eyes and a clear nasal discharge.

D   This man is showing signs of a basal skull fracture. The presenting symp-toms and signs depend on the region of skull fracture. Anterior cranial fossa fractures may present with symptoms of anosmia (loss of smell) and signs of rhinorrhoea (cerebrospinal fluid leaking through a cribriform plate injury) and periorbital ecchymosis (the classical 'raccoon eyes').

Symptoms of middle cranial fossa fracture include hearing loss and vertigo. Signs include Battle's sign (bruising behind the ear signifying temporal bone fracture), haemotympanum and cranial nerve palsies (V, VI, VII, VIII are at risk).

Posterior cranial fossa involvement may be associated with cranial nerve palsies (IX, X, XI at risk) and brainstem compression signs.

A 25-year-old was involved in a high-speed road traffic accident 48 hours ago. He has been comatosed since the injury. There are no major abnormalities on CT.

C   Diffuse axonal injury (DAI) arises from the significant shearing forces associated with acceleration–deceleration and twisting brain injury. The initial pathology is associated with the mechanical tearing of the axons, but there is also secondary brain injury later due to the initiation of biochemical cascades (associated with calcium influx).

DAI carries a poor prognosis and is associated with a persistent vegetative state. CT may show evidence of multiple cerebral contusions or may be normal. MRI is more sensitive at detecting DAI.

27 Hepatomegaly

ANSWERS: 1E, 2C, 3H, 4J

A 65-year-old man with a history of previous hepatitis B infection presents with a craggy mass in the right upper quadrant.

E   Chronic infection with hepatitis B and C is a risk factor for the development of hepatocellular carcinoma. The mechanism is unclear but there is evidence for a direct hepatocarcinogenic effect of viral infection. Other risk factors include conditions associated with liver cirrhosis and exposure to aflatoxin. There is also a recognized higher incidence of hepatocellular carcinoma in patients with type 2 diabetes mellitus.

A 42-year-old farmer presents with a history of shortness of breath and abdominal pain. Clinical examination shows enlargement of the liver. Ultrasound reveals numerous cystic lesions within the liver.

C   Hydatid disease or echinococcosis is a parasitic disease that affects both humans and mammals, e.g. sheep, dogs, horses. The clinical presentation derives from the life cycle of the parasite. The adult worm lives in the intestinal wall of the definitive host (usually dog, sheep etc). The host parasite releases eggs that are passed in the faeces of the definitive host. The egg is then ingested by an intermediate host e.g. human via contact with the animal faeces. The egg then hatches in the small intestine of the intermediate host and releases an oncosphere that invades the intestinal wall. This can lead to haematogenous spread into different organs, in particular the liver and lungs. The oncosphere develops into a cyst within these organs. The cyst enlarges creating protoscolices and daughter cysts within the cyst. A definitive host (e.g. dog) can become infected after ingesting the cyst-containing organs of the infected intermediate host (e.g. sheep). The protoscolices in the infected food can then attach to the intestinal wall, develop into adult worms and continue the cycle.

Live hydatid lung cysts are often asymptomatic but may grow to cause shortness of breath and abdominal pain. Rupture of cysts can lead to a massive immune reaction including anaphylactic shock.

A 26-year-old man presents with significant bilateral cervical lymphadenopathy, shortness of breath and marked hepatosplenomegaly. CT reveals extensive mediastinal, para-aortic and pelvic lymphadenopathy and confirms moderate enlargement of the liver and spleen.

H Lymphoma is the most common haematological malignancy. Diffuse large B-cell lymphoma makes up the majority of cases in adults. Symptoms may include weight loss, night sweats and fevers. Mediastinal lymphadenopathy may result in a persistent cough or shortness of breath. Hepatosplenomegaly is a recognized finding in lymphoma and may be the only finding in indolent cases.

A 31-year-old pregnant woman presents with a history of upper abdominal pain and jaundice. Examination of the abdomen reveals hepatomegaly and ascites.

J Budd–Chiari syndrome is caused by hepatic vein obstruction. Risk factors include pregnancy, polycythaemia vera, oral contraceptive pill, tendencies towards thrombosis (e.g. protein C deficiency, compression of the hepatic vein by tumour). The acute syndrome presents with severe upper abdominal pain, hepatomegaly, jaundice and ascites. Treatment includes symptomatic management e.g. sodium restriction and diuretics for ascites and anticoagulation. Shunts to divert blood around the obstruction e.g. transjugular intrahepatic portosystemic shunt (TIPS) may also be used.

28 Bleeding diatheses

ANSWERS: 1C, 2A, 3G, 4I

A 75-year-old woman with a previous history of stroke on the waiting list for laparascopic cholecystectomy is found to bruise easily.

C Given that there is a history of stroke it is likely that the patient is on secondary prevention anti-thrombotic therapy. Every stroke patient with a history of persistent or paroxysmal AF will be started on anticoagulation therapy unless this is contraindicated. Warfarin therapy will need to be discontinued for a few days before surgery to allow the INR to reduce to a safe level to prevent excessive perioperative and postoperative haemorrhage. Depending upon a risk assessment of thrombotic potential the patient may need postoperative cover with a low molecular weight heparin subcutaneously.

A 38-year-old on the intensive care unit with sepsis following bowel surgery is found to have bleeding from the wound site. Prothrombin time (PT), and activated partial thromboplastin time (APTT) are markedly prolonged.

A   Disseminated intravascular coagulopathy (DIC) is a pathological activation of the coagulation cascade and dysregulation of fibrinolysis with resultant widespread clotting and bleeding. Endothelial cell injury following sepsis with release of inflammatory cytokines like interleukin 1 and tumour necrosis factor promotes the release of tissue factor that is a prominent mediator of DIC. The primary treatment involves treating the underlying cause (usually sepsis).

A 17-year-old woman presents with recurrent persistent epistaxes. There is a family history of the problem and her father required numerous operations to treat the nose bleeds.

G   Hereditary haemorrhagic telangiectasia is an autosomal dominant condition which is associated with abnormal blood vessel formation particularly in the skin and mucous membranes of the nose/gastrointestinal tract. There is also a higher incidence of arterio-venous malformations in larger organs particularly the lung, liver and brain. Epistaxes may be difficult to manage as traditional packing often traumatizes the nasal lining further exacerbating the bleeding. Laser therapy to the septum is often effective but usually requires several treatments to keep symptoms at bay. In more severe cases more extensive surgery may be required including the use of skin grafts or even sealing the nostril completely.

A 9-year-old boy is referred to the orthopaedic department with a haemarthrosis of the right knee following a minor accident in the playground.

I   Factor VIII deficiency is more commonly known as haemophilia A. It is an X-linked recessive condition and is therefore much more common in males. The lack of factor VIII results in impaired fibrin formation and therefore greatly prolonged bleeding times. Minor trauma may be associated with significant bleeding. Haemarthrosis may result in damage to the joint and can increase the risk of arthritis developing later in life. The availability of recombinant factor VIII means that many patients can enjoy a near normal quality of life.

29 Congenital heart disease

ANSWERS: 1G, 2A, 3D, 4I

A 55-year-old patient is referred to the cardiothoracic surgeons with episodes of chest pain and syncope. On examination there is a marked ejection systolic murmur.

G   Bicuspid aortic valve is caused by fusion of two aortic valve leaflets during development resulting in a valve which is bicuspid rather than the normal tricuspid configuration. During childhood and early adulthood it is often asymptomatic. However, progressive calcification with age may lead to worsening aortic stenosis. This gives rise to the classic ejection systolic murmur.

In mild cases the degree of stenosis can be monitored but symptomatic cases/severe stenosis requires aortic valve replacement surgery.

A 3-month-old baby is referred with failure to thrive and episodes of cyanosis. On examination there is marked clubbing of the fingers and toes.

A Tetralogy of Fallot refers to the combination of pulmonary infundibular stenosis, overriding aorta, ventricular septal defect (VSD) and right ventricular hypertrophy. The combination of these abnormalities results in mixing of oxygenated and deoxygenated blood in the left ventricle (due to the VSD) and a right to left shunt because of the pulmonary outflow obstruction. There is a loss of oxygen saturation which may result in episodes of cyanosis depending upon the degree of anatomical abnormality. The child may have more general symptoms like failing to thrive and exertional dyspnoea.

The original palliative procedure was the Blalock–Thomas–Taussig shunt which involved forming an anastomosis between the subclavian and pulmonary artery. Advances in cardiothoracic and anaesthetic bypass techniques have now allowed the ability to carry out a total surgical repair.

A 34-year-old male is found to have an early diastolic murmur. On examination he is tall and slim with hypermobile joints. His father died in his early forties.

D Marfan syndrome is an autosomal dominant genetic disorder of connective tissue. In particular there is defective production of the protein fibrillin-1. Cardiovascular complications include mitral/aortic valve prolapse giving rise to regurgitation, aortic dilatation/aneurysm formation and an increased risk of aortic dissection. The latter is often fatal even when recognized. The presence of aortic root dilatation is now an important criterion in making the diagnosis of Marfan syndrome. The characteristic skeletal features include a tall slim physique, arachnodactyly (spindling of fingers) and hypermobile joints. There may also be abnormalities of the chest e.g. pectus excavatum. The decision to operate depends upon the severity of the aortic regurgitation but is strongly indicated where the aortic root is 4.5 cm in the patient with Marfan syndrome regardless of the severity of regurgitation symptoms.

A 26-year-old girl with Turner syndrome presents with raised blood pressure. On examination the femoral pulses are diminished.

I Aortic coarctation is a pathological narrowing of the aorta that usually occurs just distal to the origin of the left subclavian artery. It occurs more commonly in men but is associated with Turner syndrome. Patients may present with heart failure or problems resulting from reduced arterial perfusion to the lower half of the body (hence the diminished femoral pulses). The diagnosis is usually made during assessment of hypertension or as an incidental finding. In the first instance treatment involves managing the resulting hypertension. Surgical options include resection with end to end anastomosis, subclavian flap aortoplasty, balloon angioplasty and endovascular stenting.

30 Eponymous surgical procedures

ANSWERS: 1I, 2H, 3C, 4A

A patient requiring surgery for a thyroglossal cyst.

I Walter Ellis Sistrunk described an operation for thyroglossal cyst excision in 1920. It involves removing the cyst and a core of tissue surrounding the tract and following it up to the central portion of the hyoid bone which is excised. Any further tract is followed and excised up to the foramen caecum. Taking the extra tissue either side of the tract as a central neck dissection significantly reduces the risk of recurrent cyst formation.

A patient with a tumour in the head of the pancreas.

H Allen Whipple was an American surgeon who described his procedure in the 1930s. The operation involves removing the head of the pancreas, part of the bile duct, gallbladder and duodenum. Indications for the procedure include carcinoma of the head of pancreas, cholangiocarcinoma and ampullary tumours.

A patient with a symptomatic paraoesophageal hiatus hernia.

C A Nissen's fundoplication involves wrapping/plicating the gastric fundus around the inferior part of the oesophagus which restores the function of the lower oesophageal sphincter. This prevents the reflux of gastric acid and/or the sliding of the fundus through the enlarged oesophageal hiatus in the diaphragm. This procedure is now more commonly performed via a laparascopic technique or robot-assisted surgery.

A child with severe pyloric stenosis.

A Ramstedt's procedure is the definitive treatment for severe pyloric stenosis. Traditionally it was an open procedure which involved making a single incision through the circular and longitudinal muscles of the pylorus to relieve the stenosis. It is now more commonly performed via a laparascopic technique as this is associated with a shorter time to begin full enteral feeding and a shorter hospital stay.

31 Clinical trials

ANSWERS 1I, 2C, 3E, 4D

The study associated with the highest level of evidence.

I   A systematic review or meta-analysis of randomized controlled trials is deemed to provide level Ia evidence which provides the strongest evidence from the options above. The Centre for Evidence Based Medicine in Oxford gives an up-to-date précis of the levels of evidence for studies depending upon whether they involve therapy, diagnosis or prognosis. In basic terms, for therapy studies the below applies:

Ia	Systematic review/meta-analysis randomized controlled trials
Ib	Individual randomized controlled trial/cohort study
IIa	Systematic review of cohort studies
IIb	Individual cohort study
IIc	Ecological study, 'outcomes research'
IIIa	Systematic review case control studies
IIIb	Single case control study
IV	Case series
V	Expert opinion

Individuals with varying degrees of sunlight exposure are followed up for many years and observed for the incidence of skin cancer.

C   Cohort studies are particularly good at determining the incidence and natural history of a condition. In a prospective cohort study a 'cohort' of patients is selected that do not have a particular disease/condition and then are monitored over time with regard to specific variables to see if they develop the outcome of interest. Cohort studies may also be retrospective by analysing data already collected for other purposes. The advantage of a cohort study is that you can investigate several variables. Depending upon the study it may also be possible to establish causation.

A notes review of 100 people treated with transoral laser therapy is used to measure the incidence of dry mouth.

E   A case series is a descriptive study that involves selecting a group of cases to observe the effect of a single exposure with a particular outcome measure. It tends to be useful when the disease under investigation is uncommon and when it is caused by a single kind of exposure.

A group of schoolboys is given a questionnaire survey to find out the number that had a history of appendicectomy.

D   A cross sectional study is particularly useful in determining prevalence of a condition. It involves assessing the outcome of interest at one point in time. Questionnaires are commonly used in cross sectional studies. The advantage of a cross sectional study is that it is cheap, quick and can be used to study multiple outcomes. However, it cannot be used to establish causation.

SECTION 2: ORTHOPAEDIC SURGERY

QUESTIONS

32 Hand conditions

A	Dupuytren's contracture	G	ganglion
B	trigger finger	H	scaphoid fracture
C	carpal tunnel syndrome	I	osteosarcoma
D	ulnar collateral ligament injury	J	osteoarthritis of first MCP
E	ulnar nerve injury	K	radial nerve injury
F	De Quervain's stenosing tenovaginitis	L	fibrous dysplasia

For each clinical scenario below give the most likely cause for the clinical findings. Each option may be used only once.

1   A 74-year-old man presents with inability to extend the ring finger. On examination his ring finger is locked in flexion but can be released with manipulation.

2   A 42-year-old woman presents with a firm swelling over the dorsum of the wrist. It has been fluctuating in size and causes discomfort when typing.

3   A 36-year-old woman presents with pain over the radial aspect of the wrist. On examination pain is elicited by forced adduction and flexion of the thumb.

4   A 24-year-old presents with pain and swelling over the base of thumb following a skiing accident. His grip is weak.

ANSWERS: see page 91

33 Arthritis

A	psoriatic arthritis	H	Reiter's syndrome
B	discoid lupus erythematosus	I	Sjögren's syndrome
C	rheumatoid arthritis	J	ankylosing spondylosis
D	polymyalgia rheumatica	K	septic arthritis
E	systemic lupus erythematosus	L	gout
F	cervical spondylosis	M	osteoporosis
G	lumbar spondylosis	N	osteoarthritis

For each clinical scenario below give the most likely cause for the clinical findings. Each option may be used only once.

1   A 54-year-old woman presents to her GP with pain and swelling affecting her fingers, wrists, knees and feet. On examination there are signs of ulnar deviation and subluxation at the MCP joints. There are mild effusions over the painful joints and they are warm on palpation. She suggests that the symptoms are worse in the morning.

2   A 65-year-old woman complains of pain in her knees particularly on movement that is worst at the end of the day. The knees are swollen but there is no obvious effusion/warmth over the joint. Examination reveals marked reduction in flexion of both knees. X-rays show loss of joint space and subchondral cysts.

3   A 30-year-old woman complains of joint pain in her hands and feet. Chest x-ray shows reduced lung volumes.

4   A 22-year-old man presents with an acute arthritis of the left knee, dysuria and bilateral conjunctivitis. He has recently suffered from gastroenteritis.

5   A 45-year-old woman presents with bilateral painful deformed distal interphalangeal joints. Examination reveals discoloration and onycholysis of the nails.

ANSWERS: see page 92

34 Joint pain

A	psoriatic arthritis	H	Reiter's syndrome
B	polymyositis	I	osteosarcoma
C	rheumatoid arthritis	J	pseudogout
D	polymyalgia rheumatica	K	septic arthritis
E	systemic lupus erythematosus	L	gout
F	haemarthrosis	M	osteoporosis
G	lumbar spondylosis			

For each clinical scenario below give the most likely cause for the clinical findings. Each option may be used only once.

1   A 64-year-old patient who has recently been started on medication for hypertension presents with a very painful, hot, swollen metatarsophalangeal joint.

2   A 12-year-old haemophiliac presents to A&E with severe pain after falling over and banging his right knee.

3   A 55-year-old man presents to A&E with fever and an exquisitely painful right knee. On examination his right knee is red, hot and swollen. Purulent fluid is aspirated from the joint.

4   A 60-year-old woman presents with a painful swollen knee. X-ray shows chondrocalcinosis and joint aspiration reveals the presence of weakly positive birefringent crystals.

5   A 65-year-old woman presents with a 1-month history of pain and stiffness in her shoulders, worse in the mornings. She says she was treated in hospital last year for headache and jaw pain.

ANSWERS: see page 93

35 Pain in the hip

A	slipped upper femoral epiphysis	H	septic arthritis
B	osteoarthritis	I	fractured sacroiliac joint
C	congenital dislocation of hip	J	fractured neck of femur
D	fractured pubic ramus	K	Charcot joint
E	transient synovitis	L	idiopathic growth retardation
F	tuberculous arthritis	M	Perthes' disease
G	rheumatoid arthritis		

For each clinical scenario below give the most likely cause for the clinical findings. Each option may be used only once.

1   An obese 12-year-old boy presents with pain in his right hip. On examination the hip is flexed, abducted and externally rotated. His mother has suffered from tuberculosis in the past.

2   A 6-year-old boy presents with a pain in the hip and a limp. All movements at the hip are limited. X-ray shows decrease in size of the femoral head with patchy density.

3   A 2-year-old girl presents to the orthopaedic clinic with a waddling gait. Her mother says that there has been a delay in walking. On examination there is an extra crease on the left thigh.

4   An 80-year-old woman presents to A&E following a fall. On examination the left hip is shortened, externally rotated and all movements are painful.

5   An 8-year-old boy presents to A&E with a marked limp and pain in the right hip which resolves within 48 hours. X-rays show no abnormality at the hip or other joint involvement. Bone scan 2 weeks later is also normal.

ANSWERS: see page 94

36 Back pain

A	Paget's disease	G	myeloma
B	polymyositis	H	rheumatoid arthritis
C	Scheuermann's disease	I	Pott's disease
D	vertebral disc prolapse	J	spinal stenosis
E	osteomyelitis	K	ankylosing spondylitis
F	Reiter's disease		

For each clinical scenario below give the most likely cause for the clinical findings. Each option may be used only once.

1 A 22-year-old man complains of stiffness in the lower back and buttock pain that is relieved by exercise. He also suffers from bouts of painful red eye. ESR is raised. X-ray shows blurring of the upper vertebral rims of the lumbar spine.

2 A 60-year-old woman presents with constant backache. ESR and serum calcium are markedly elevated.

3 A 65-year-old man with osteoarthritis complains of back pain, worse on walking, along with aching and heaviness in both legs that forces him to stop walking. Pain is relieved slowly after rest or leaning forward.

4 A 13-year-old girl complains of backache and fatigue. Her mother has noticed that she is becoming increasingly round-shouldered. On examination, she has a smooth thoracic kyphosis. X-ray shows wedge-shaped vertebral bodies in the thoracic spine.

5 A 35-year-old tourist complains of severe back pain with inability to straighten up after lifting a suitcase yesterday. He now presents with weakness of big toe extension and loss of sensation on the outer side of the calf.

ANSWERS: see page 96

37 Complications of fractures

A	compartment syndrome	G	delayed union
B	osteoporosis	H	Sudeck's atrophy
C	pneumothorax	I	malunion
D	ulnar nerve injury	J	myositis ossificans
E	pulmonary embolus	K	haemarthrosis
F	median nerve injury	L	radial nerve injury

For each clinical scenario below give the most likely cause for the clinical findings. Each option may be used only once.

1   A 25-year-old man presents with a blue right arm with absent radial pulse and painful passive finger extension following a supracondylar fracture of humerus.

2   A 40-year-old woman presents 5 weeks after a radial fracture with a painful swollen hand. The hand is cold and cyanosed with heightened temperature sensitivity.

3   A 70-year-old woman complains of right-sided pleuritic chest pain 10 days after a fractured neck of femur.

4   A 60-year-old woman complains of pain, swelling and reduced mobility 4 months after suffering a fractured tibia. X-ray shows absence of callus at the fracture site.

5   A 65-year-old woman who falls on her outstretched arm has weakness in wrist extension.

ANSWERS: see page 97

38 Management of fractures

A skin traction
B collar and cuff sling
C broad arm sling
D hip spica
E gallows traction
F internal fixation
G complete bed rest and
   immobilization

H manipulation under local
   anaesthesia and backslab
I long thumb spica cast
J analgesia + encourage
   weight-bearing

For each clinical scenario below suggest the most appropriate management. Each option may be used only once.

1 A 24-year-old man presents with a swollen painful hand after falling over playing squash. X-ray reveals a scaphoid fracture.

2 A 75-year-old woman presents to A&E with groin pain and inability to bear weight following a fall. X-ray reveals an undisplaced fracture of the superior pubic ramus.

3 A 65-year-old woman presents with a displaced extracapsular fractured neck of femur.

4 A 35-year-old woman presents after a fall on an outstretched arm. X-ray shows a minimally displaced surgical neck fracture of the right humerus.

5 A 75-year-old woman presents to A&E with a displaced Colles fracture.

ANSWERS: see page 98

39 Fall on the outstretched hand

A	Colles fracture	G	Galeazzi fracture
B	scapular fracture	H	fracture of clavicle
C	posterior dislocation of shoulder	I	Monteggia fracture
D	olecranon fracture	J	supracondylar fracture
E	anterior dislocation of shoulder	K	fractured humeral shaft
F	scaphoid fracture	L	Smith's fracture

For each clinical scenario below suggest the most likely injury that has resulted. Each option may be used only once.

1 A 24-year-old woman presents with pain on wrist movements after falling on her hand. On examination there is tenderness and swelling in the anatomical snuff box.

2 A 68-year-old woman presents with a fracture of the distal radius with dorsal displacement of the distal fragment after a fall.

3 A 7-year-old boy presents with a swollen painful elbow following a fall. He is unable to move the arm due to pain.

4 A 19-year-old rugby player falls on a backward stretched hand and presents with loss of shoulder contour and absent sensation in the military badge area below the shoulder.

5 A 40-year-old woman presents after a fall on an outstretched hand, with pain in the upper arm and a wrist drop.

ANSWERS: see page 99

40 Shoulder conditions

A	ruptured long head of biceps	G	posterior dislocation of shoulder
B	Sprengel's shoulder	H	anterior dislocation of shoulder
C	tendonitis of long head of biceps	I	fracture of clavicle
D	osteoarthritis	J	fractured neck of humerus
E	impingement syndrome	K	adhesive capsulitis
F	rheumatoid arthritis	L	fractured scapula

For each clinical scenario below give the most likely cause for the clinical findings. Each option may be used only once.

1   A 21-year-old woman presents with a very painful shoulder locked in adduction and internal rotation following an epileptic fit.

2   A 55-year-old man complains of shoulder pain aggravated in abduction of the arm between 60° and 120°.

3   A 30-year-old bodybuilder presents with a painful shoulder after weightlifting. Flexing his elbow reveals a prominent lump in the upper arm.

4   A 50-year-old man complains of a 9-month history of stiffness in the shoulder. The shoulder was originally extremely painful but now only the stiffness remains.

5   A 65-year-old woman presents with shoulder pain and restricted movement in all directions. X-ray shows reduced joint space and subchondral sclerosis.

ANSWERS: see page 100

41 Knee conditions

A	genu varum	G	dislocation of patella
B	collateral ligament rupture	H	genu valgum
C	suprapatellar bursitis	I	osteoarthritis
D	Baker's cyst	J	anterior cruciate ligament tear
E	prepatellar bursitis	K	meniscal cyst
F	meniscal tear	L	Osgood–Schlatter disease

For each clinical scenario below give the most likely cause for the clinical findings. Each option may be used only once.

1   A 22-year-old figure-skater presents with a painful locked knee with limited extension following a twisting injury.

2   A 24-year-old footballer presents with a painful knee after landing awkwardly and twisting his knee after a header. With the quadriceps relaxed, there is excessive anterior glide of the tibia on the femur.

3   A 14-year-old girl successfully treated for rickets 3 years ago shows bow-legged deformity.

4   A 16-year-old boy complains of a painful knee during exercise and a tender lump over the tibial tuberosity.

5   A 50-year-old carpet layer presents with a swelling directly over the patella. The joint feels stable and there is no effusion.

ANSWERS: see page 101

42 Management of painful joints

A	exercise and physiotherapy	H	flucloxacillin + benzylpenicillin i.v.
B	paracetamol		
C	allopurinol	I	hydrocortisone i.v.
D	colchicine	J	sulphasalazine
E	high-dose aspirin	K	ibuprofen
F	oral penicillin	L	methotrexate
G	oral prednisolone		

For each clinical scenario below suggest the most appropriate management. Each option may be used only once.

1 A 24-year-old man presented with lower back pain and stiffness that was worse in the morning. He has developed a thoracic kyphosis and has a hyperextended neck.

2 An 80-year-old man with a 30-year history of rheumatoid arthritis presents to A&E with fever and pain in the right knee. On examination his right knee is red, hot and swollen. Aspirated synovial fluid is frankly purulent.

3 A 65-year-old woman recently diagnosed with osteoarthritis requires medication for night pain.

4 A 64-year-old woman who has been successfully treated for acute gout requires prophylactic medication.

5 A 65-year-old woman with painful shoulders due to polymyalgia rheumatica.

ANSWERS: see page 102

43 Foot conditions

A	pes planus	G	claw toe
B	plantar fasciitis	H	hammer toe
C	osteomyelitis	I	deltoid ligament injury
D	hallux rigidus	J	Morton's neuroma
E	pes cavus	K	osteochondroma
F	march fracture	L	Achilles heel rupture

For each clinical scenario below give the most likely cause for the clinical findings. Each option may be used only once.

1   A 32-year-old marathon runner presents with persistent pain over the dorsum of the foot on weight-bearing.

2   A 62-year-old man presents with persistent pain over the left big toe. On examination there is swelling and decreased range of movement over the first metatarsophalangeal joint.

3   A 24-year-old man presents with pain in his right heel that is worse in the morning. On examination there is pain on passive dorsiflexion of the toes and when walking on tip-toes.

4   A 50-year-old woman complains of pain over the dorsal aspect of the PIP joint of the second toe. On examination there is a flexion deformity of the PIP with hyperextension at the DIP joint.

ANSWERS: see page 103

44 Lower limb nerve lesion

A   tibial nerve
B   common peroneal nerve
C   obturator nerve
D   femoral nerve
E   saphenous nerve
F   ilioinguinal nerve

G   iliohypogastric nerve
H   genitofemoral nerve
I   superior gluteal nerve
J   sciatic nerve
K   pudendal nerve

Choose the most likely location of the lesion that gives rise to the symptoms below. Each option may be used only once.

1   A 22-year-old footballer complains of weakness of dorsiflexion of the right foot after suffering an injury to the side of the knee.

2   A 75-year-old patient presents with a profound foot drop several days after a hip hemiarthroplasty for a fractured neck of femur.

3   A 38-year-old woman complains of sensation loss over the anteromedial aspect of the lower leg following varicose vein surgery.

4   A 36-year-old man is brought to A&E after suffering penetrating trauma to the right popliteal fossa. On examination there is loss of active plantar flexion and loss of sensation over the sole of the foot.

ANSWERS: see page 104

45 Upper limb nerve injury (i)

A	subscapular nerve	G	C5, C6
B	axillary nerve	H	suprascapular nerve
C	median nerve	I	T1
D	radial nerve	J	long thoracic nerve
E	musculocutaneous nerve	K	nerve to subclavius
F	ulnar nerve		

Choose the most likely location of the lesion that gives rise to the symptoms below. Each option may be used only once.

1   A 25-year-old man complains of anaesthesia over a patch on his outer upper arm following anterior dislocation of the shoulder.

2   A 63-year-old man is found to have weakness of thumb abduction following carpal tunnel release surgery.

3   A young child presents to the orthopaedic clinic with claw hand and wasting of the small muscles of the hand. There is sensory deficit to light touch along the inner and upper forearm. The only medical history of note is that the child was delivered in the breech position.

4   A 7-year-old is found to have numbness over the medial one and a half fingers after suffering a supracondylar fracture of the humerus.

ANSWERS: see page 105

46 Upper limb nerve injury (ii)

A	musculocutaneous nerve	H	radial nerve injury: wrist
B	axillary nerve	I	ulnar nerve injury: elbow
C	median nerve injury: wrist	J	long thoracic nerve
D	suprascapular nerve	K	radial nerve injury: axilla
E	median nerve injury: elbow	L	intercostal nerve
F	ulnar nerve injury: wrist		
G	radial nerve injury: humeral shaft		

Choose the most likely location of the lesion that gives rise to the symptoms below. Each option may be used only once.

1 A 35-year-old patient is brought to A&E following a road traffic accident. She has suffered multiple fractures to the humerus and forearm bones. On examination there is an obvious wrist drop, loss of elbow extension and sensation loss over the first dorsal web space.

2 A 45-year-old patient is brought to A&E after being assaulted. There is significant bruising over the right upper limb. On examination there is loss of forearm pronation and the hand is noted to deviate to the ulnar side when flexing the wrist.

3 A 30-year-old rugby player presents with winging of the scapula after suffering a blow to the ribs underneath an outstretched arm.

ANSWERS: see page 106

ANSWERS

32 Hand conditions

ANSWERS: 1B, 2G, 3F, 4D

A 74-year-old man presents with inability to extend the ring finger. On examination his ring finger is locked in flexion but can be released with manipulation.

B   The finger flexor tendons usually glide smoothly under the A1 pulley of the hand. If there is thickening of the flexor tendon, or if a nodule develops, the tendon can be caught under the pulley thus locking the tendon. Forceful extension/manipulation can release the tendon with transient discomfort. This condition is known as 'trigger finger'. Management can be medical or surgical. Medical intervention involves corticosteroid injections into the flexor sheath. Surgical intervention involves surgical release of the A1 pulley which can usually be performed under local anaesthesia.

A 42-year-old woman presents with a firm swelling over the dorsum of the wrist. It has been fluctuating in size and causes discomfort when typing.

G   A ganglion is a firm, smooth, cystic lesion that is closely associated with a joint or tendon sheath. This patient presents with a lesion on the dorsum of the wrist which is the most common site (related to the scapholunate ligament of the wrist). They may cause significant anxiety due to fear of malignancy, so reassurance is an important part of management. Treatment is by excision under general anaesthetic. The patient should be warned about the risk of recurrence.

A 36-year-old woman presents with pain over the radial aspect of the wrist. On examination pain is elicited by forced adduction and flexion of the thumb.

F   Pain on forced adduction and flexion of the thumb is known as a positive Finkelstein's sign and is suggestive of stenosing tenovaginitis. This condition is caused by inflammation and thickening of the tendon sheaths of extensor pollicis brevis and abductor pollicis longus where the tendons cross the distal radius. Medical treatment involves corticosteroid injections into the tendon sheath. Surgical intervention involves splitting the tendon sheath.

A 24-year-old presents with pain and swelling over the base of thumb following a skiing accident. His grip is weak.

D   This injury was previously known as 'gamekeeper's thumb' which referred to a chronic injury to the ulnar collateral ligament caused by repetitive wringing of necks of game. Nowadays the damage to the ulnar collateral ligament is caused by an acute severe abducting force to the thumb. It is associated with ski injury due to the position of the ski-pole strap across the palm which transmits the force of injury to the thumb during a fall. With minor injuries conservative measures and physiotherapy are often sufficient. If there is complete rupture surgical intervention is indicated.

33 Arthritis

ANSWERS: 1C, 2N, 3E, 4H, 5A

A 54-year-old woman presents to her GP with pain and swelling affecting her fingers, wrists, knees and feet. On examination there are signs of ulnar deviation and subluxation at the MCP joints. There are mild effusions over the painful joints and they are warm on palpation. She suggests that the symptoms are worse in the morning.

C   Ulnar deviation and subluxation of metacarpophalangeal joints (MCPs) are signs of advanced rheumatoid disease. Swelling of the fingers (sausage-like) and MCP joint swelling are earlier signs.

A 65-year-old woman complains of pain in her knees particularly on movement that is worst at the end of the day. The knees are swollen but there is no obvious effusion/warmth over the joint. Examination reveals marked reduction in flexion of both knees. X-rays show loss of joint space and subchondral cysts.

N   The x-ray changes of osteoarthritis include loss of joint space, subchondral sclerosis, osteophytes and subchondral cyst formation. Osteophytes at the proximal and distal interphalangeal joints are called Bouchard's and Heberden's nodes respectively. Previous joint damage is a risk factor for the development of osteoarthritic disease. Simple analgesics like paracetamol should be prescribed for pain relief rather than long courses of NSAIDs (risk of GI bleeding with prolonged use).

A 30-year-old woman complains of joint pain in her hands and feet. Chest x-ray shows reduced lung volumes.

E   Systemic lupus erythematosus (SLE) is an inflammatory multisystemic disorder that is nine times more common in women than men. The joints are most often affected in a symmetrical fashion with no bony erosion (unlike rheumatoid arthritis). Rarely there may be markedly deformed joints due to joint laxity that resemble rheumatoid arthritis (Jaccoud's arthropathy).

Lung involvement occurs in up to half of patients with SLE. Manifestations include pleuritic chest pain, pleural effusions (these are common and often bilateral), acute/chronic pneumonitis and the rare 'shrinking lung syndrome'.

A 22-year-old man presents with an acute arthritis of the left knee, dysuria and bilateral conjunctivitis. He has recently suffered from gastroenteritis.

H   Reiter's disease involves a triad of urethritis, conjunctivitis and seronegative arthritis. Joint symptoms may be the presenting complaint. It is often triggered by an infection (e.g. a sexually transmitted disease or gastroenteritis). Cutaneous manifestations include keratoderma blenorrhagica, circinate balanitis and mouth ulcers. Enthesitis causing plantar fasciitis is also well recognized.

A 45-year-old woman presents with bilateral painful deformed distal interphalangeal joints. Examination reveals discoloration and onycholysis of the nails.

A   Psoriatic arthritis is one of the seronegative spondyloarthritides. It is important to remember that the skin manifestations may occur subsequent to joint involvement. The patient in the question shows a typical presentation of distal interphalangeal joint involvement with signs of nail dystrophy. Radiologically the affected joints show central erosion rather than the juxta-articular involvement that is seen in rheumatoid arthritis.

About 5 per cent of patients with psoriasis may present with marked deformity in the fingers caused by severe periarticular osteolysis. This is known as arthritis mutilans.

34 Joint pain

ANSWERS: 1L, 2F, 3K, 4J, 5D

A 64-year-old patient who has recently been started on medication for hypertension presents with a very painful, hot, swollen metatarsophalangeal joint.

L   Gout is associated with hyperuricaemia and therefore acute attacks may be precipitated by impaired excretion/increased production of uric acid. Drugs that impair the excretion of uric acid include thiazide diuretics and aspirin. States of increased cell turnover and thus increased purine turnover (e.g. myelo/lymphoproliferative states or carcinoma) can predispose to gout. Obesity, diabetes mellitus, high alcohol intake and hypertension are associated with hyperuricaemia.

A 12-year-old haemophiliac presents to A&E with severe pain after falling over and banging his right knee.

F Bleeding into the joint (haemarthrosis) may occur in all patients but is more common in those with acquired/inherited disorders of coagulation like haemophilia. Development of haemarthrosis is usually immediate (e.g. following ligamentous injury) whereas a serous effusion is usually delayed.

A 55-year-old man presents to A&E with fever and an exquisitely painful right knee. On examination his right knee is red, hot and swollen. Purulent fluid is aspirated from the joint.

K The differential diagnosis of a monoarthritis is septic arthritis, osteoarthritis, crystal-induced arthritis, trauma-related or a single joint manifestation of a multi-joint disease. Septic arthritis is a medical emergency. When a patient presents with a red and hot swollen knee, treatment for any other possible diagnosis must not be initiated before septic arthritis is excluded. The joint space should be aspirated and the fluid sent for urgent Gram staining and culture as soon as possible. Microscopy will reveal the presence of crystals if the diagnosis is gout/pseudogout.

A 60-year-old woman presents with a painful swollen knee. X-ray shows chondrocalcinosis and joint aspiration reveals the presence of weakly positive birefringent crystals.

J Pseudogout refers to the acute synovitis caused by the deposition of calcium pyrophosphate crystals into a joint. The knee and the wrist are the two most commonly affected sites. Diagnosis is made by detection of crystals that are weakly positively birefringent in plane polarized light. Risk factors include hypovolaemia, hyperparathyroidism, diabetes, haemochromatosis, acromegaly and any another pre-existing arthritis.

A 65-year-old woman presents with a 1-month history of pain and stiffness in her shoulders, worse in the mornings. She says she was treated in hospital last year for headache and jaw pain.

D Polymyalgia rheumatica is associated with giant cell arteritis and is very rare under the age of 50 years. Patients also often complain of fatigue and depression. It is typically associated with a high ESR. Oral prednisolone is the treatment of choice.

35 Pain in the hip

ANSWERS: 1A, 2M, 3C, 4J, 5E

An obese 12-year-old boy presents with pain in his right hip. On examination the hip is flexed, abducted and externally rotated. His mother has suffered from tuberculosis in the past.

A   This is a classical presentation of slipped upper femoral epiphysis and the previous history of TB in the mother is not significant. The patient is obese and presents with limping and pain in the groin, thigh or knee. This condition is most common in the 10- to 16-year age group. A lateral x-ray is required to show the abnormality more clearly.

Tuberculous arthritis is very rare in the UK, affecting mostly the elderly and infants.

A 6-year-old boy presents with a pain in the hip and a limp. All movements at the hip are limited. X-ray shows decrease in size of the femoral head with patchy density.

M   Perthes' disease is osteochondritis of the femoral head and classically affects children in a younger age group compared to slipped upper femoral epiphysis (around 3–11 years). It is around four times more common in males. The younger the patient, the better the prognosis. In many cases, rest is sufficient treatment. In severe disease, surgery may be indicated.

A 2-year-old girl presents to the orthopaedic clinic with a waddling gait. Her mother says that there has been a delay in walking. On examination there is an extra crease on the left thigh.

C   Congenital dislocation of the hip (CDH) is around six times more common in females and is more common after breech delivery. The Ortolani test and Barlow's manoeuvre are performed to identify this condition which is bilateral in about a third of cases. In Ortolani's test the examiner holds the baby's thighs with the thumbs placed medially and the fingers resting on the greater trochanters. The examiner flexes the hips to 90° and gently abducts to almost 90°. In CDH this movement is difficult and if pressure is applied to the greater trochanter there is an audible click as the dislocation reduces. Barlow's test involves the examiner grasping the upper thigh with the thumb placed in the groin and attempting to lever the femoral head in and out of the acetabulum as he/she abducts and adducts the thigh. Ultrasound screening is more commonly used now to diagnose and monitor this condition.

An 80-year-old woman presents to A&E following a fall. On exami-nation the left hip is shortened, externally rotated and all movements are painful.

J   The classical deformity of the fractured neck of femur (NOF) is limb shortening with external rotation of the leg. As a result of the fracture the pull of the iliopsoas twists the femur into external rotation rather than simply flexing the hip joint. The pull of the short gluteal muscles shortens the leg. There may be particular tenderness over the anterior and lateral aspects of the hip joint.

NOF fractures can be broadly described as *intracapsular* or *extracapsular*. The former are more likely to disrupt the blood supply to the femoral head and can be treated by cannulated screws or joint replacement if very displaced or if the patient is elderly and needs to fully weight-bear immediately after surgery.

An 8-year-old boy presents to A&E with a marked limp and pain in the right hip which resolves within 48 hours. X-rays show no abnormality at the hip or other joint involvement. Bone scan 2 weeks later is also normal.

E   The patient must have a normal x-ray for the diagnosis to be made. This condition is also known as 'irritable hip'. Transient synovitis is a diagnosis of exclusion; i.e. the diagnosis is made only when all other possible diagnoses are eliminated.

36 Back pain

ANSWERS: 1K, 2G, 3J, 4C, 5D

A 22-year-old man complains of stiffness in the lower back and buttock pain that is relieved by exercise. He also suffers from bouts of painful red eye. ESR is raised. X-ray shows blurring of the upper vertebral rims of the lumbar spine.

K   This man's buttock pain is caused by sacroiliitis. Blurring of the vertebral rims is an early sign on x-ray, resulting from enthesitis at the insertion of intervertebral ligaments. Later, persistent enthesitis leads to the formation of bony spurs called syndesmophytes.

A 60-year-old woman presents with constant backache. ESR and serum calcium are markedly elevated.

G   Back pain is common in the elderly and the cause is often benign. However, constant symptoms, raised ESR and raised serum calcium raises the suspicion of underlying myeloma.

A 65-year-old man with osteoarthritis complains of back pain, worse on walking, along with aching and heaviness in both legs that forces him to stop walking. Pain is relieved slowly after rest or leaning forward.

J   This is a classical description of spinal claudication (leaning forward opens the spinal canal and relieves pain). In vascular claudication the pain is quickly relieved upon rest whereas the relief from pain occurs later in spinal claudication. Operative decompression can be very successful in treating symptoms of pain in patients who are severely affected.

A 13-year-old girl complains of backache and fatigue. Her mother has noticed that she is becoming increasingly round-shouldered.

On examination, she has a smooth thoracic kyphosis. X-ray shows wedge-shaped vertebral bodies in the thoracic spine.

C   Scheuermann's disease is a rare condition that typically affects teenagers. There is abnormal ossification of ring epiphyses of thoracic vertebrae. The deforming forces are greatest at the anterior border of the vertebrae, giving rise to the described wedge-shaped vertebral bodies (i.e. narrower anteriorly). Management depends on the degree of kyphosis and ranges from back strengthening exercises and postural training in those mildly affected to operative correction and fusion in those with severe kyphosis.

A 35-year-old tourist complains of severe back pain with inability to straighten up after lifting a suitcase yesterday. He now presents with weakness of big toe extension and loss of sensation on the outer side of the calf.

D   This man is showing symptoms of nerve compression at the L5 level and MRI is indicated for confirmation of diagnosis and assessment of level/degree of compression. Symptoms can sometimes be managed in the early stages by limited intervention (e.g. physiotherapy, painkillers and epidural injection), but decompression surgery is the definitive management strategy if conservative measures fail.

37 Complications of fractures

ANSWERS: 1A, 2H, 3E, 4G, 5L

A 25-year-old man presents with a blue right arm with absent radial pulse and painful passive finger extension following a supracondylar fracture of humerus.

A   Fracture can lead to ischaemia in the distal limb by direct injury to the blood vessel or by the effect of oedema increasing the pressure within the osteofascial compartment which limits perfusion. In compartment syndrome, the increased pressure can lead to profound ischaemia with necrosis of muscle and nerve tissue. This is a surgical emergency requiring prompt decompression by open fasciotomy. Once muscle tissue dies it is replaced by inelastic fibrous tissue giving rise to the complication of Volkmann's ischaemic contracture.

A 40-year-old woman presents 5 weeks after a radial fracture with a painful swollen hand. The hand is cold and cyanosed with heightened temperature sensitivity.

H   This condition is now known as 'complex regional pain syndrome type 1'. The pain and swelling is close to but not exactly at the area of injury. The skin may be oedematous and there may be altered sweat production. Its aetiology is unknown.

A 70-year-old woman complains of right-sided pleuritic chest pain 10 days after a fractured neck of femur.

E   Pleuritic chest pain following orthopaedic/pelvic surgery should invoke strong suspicion of pulmonary embolus.

A 60-year-old woman complains of pain, swelling and reduced mobility 4 months after suffering a fractured tibia. X-ray shows absence of callus at the fracture site.

G   Absence of callus at the fracture site implies delayed union. Malunion is diagnosed if the fracture heals with non-anatomical alignment.

A 65-year-old woman who falls on her outstretched arm has weakness in wrist extension.

L   The radial nerve supplies motor innervation to the extensors of the wrist. Look out for signs of radial nerve injury following fracture/dislocation of the elbow, fracture of the humerus, shoulder dislocation and injury to the brachial plexus/axillary region.

38 Management of fractures

ANSWERS: 1I, 2J, 3F, 4B, 5H

A 24-year-old man presents with a swollen painful hand after falling over playing squash. X-ray reveals a scaphoid fracture.

I   The wrist is held in dorsiflexion. A plaster cast from the wrist to above the knuckle provides insufficient support. Internal fixation is sometimes required with displaced/non-healing fractures.

A 75-year-old woman presents to A&E with groin pain and inability to bear weight following a fall. X-ray reveals an undisplaced fracture of the superior pubic ramus.

J   The pubic rami are not required for structural support when walking, so weight-bearing should be encouraged once the patient's pain has been suitably managed. Bed rest is associated with morbidity and complications such as deep vein thrombosis/pulmonary embolus and pressure sores and is not required in normally mobile patients with a pubic ramus fracture.

A 65-year-old woman presents with a displaced extracapsular fractured neck of femur.

F   This is the management of choice. Mobilization can begin immediately as internal fixation (e.g. dynamic hip screw) holds a fracture very securely.

A 35-year-old woman presents after a fall on an outstretched arm. X-ray shows a minimally displaced surgical neck fracture of the right humerus.

B   The aim of a sling is to use the gravitational force of the arm/forearm to reduce and/or hold the fracture. A collar and cuff sling permits gravity to help realign a humeral fracture, whereas a broad arm sling is more useful for helping to realign a fractured clavicle.

A 75-year-old woman presents to A&E with a displaced Colles fracture.

H   Manipulation of the fracture with a haematoma block should be attempted. The moulded cast is applied with three-point fixation from just below the elbow to the palm of the hand with the wrist slightly flexed and in mild ulnar deviation. An x-ray after reduction should be obtained to ensure that there is a satisfactory position.

39 Fall on the outstretched hand

ANSWERS: 1F, 2A, 3J, 4E, 5K

A 24-year-old woman presents with pain on wrist movements after falling on her hand. On examination there is tenderness and swelling in the anatomical snuff box.

F   The anatomical snuff box (ASB) is a triangular depression best seen when the thumb is extended. It is bounded anteriorly by the tendons of the abductor pollicis longus and extensor pollicis brevis and posteriorly by the tendon of the extensor pollicis longus. The scaphoid and trapezium lie at the base of the ASB. The radial styloid process and the base of the first metacarpal can be felt proximally and distally to the floor respectively. The radial artery and a superficial branch of the radial nerve cross the ASB.

Pain and swelling at the ASB following injury to the arm/hand suggests fracture of the scaphoid. If there is high index of suspicion for a fractured scaphoid but no positive x-ray findings, a plaster cast may be applied and an x-ray repeated 2 weeks later (the fracture may become clearer later). Alternatively, bone scans or MRI scans will reveal the injury.

A 68-year-old woman presents with a fracture of the distal radius with dorsal displacement of the distal fragment after a fall.

A   A displaced Colles fracture is sometimes described as exhibiting a 'dinner-fork' deformity. This injury is more common in older women where osteoporosis has increased the susceptibility to fracture. A Smith's fracture is a form of 'reverse' Colles fracture where the radial fragment is angled in a palmar direction. Smith's fractures are less common and often unstable, requiring internal fixation.

A 7-year-old boy presents with a swollen painful elbow following a fall. He is unable to move the arm due to pain.

J   This injury is more common in children following a fall on the outstretched hand. It is imperative to look for any signs of damage to the brachial artery. The elbow should be kept extended to avoid arterial damage. Displaced fractures are surgical emergencies and treated by reduction under general anaesthesia.

A 19-year-old rugby player falls on a backward stretched hand and presents with loss of shoulder contour and absent sensation in the military badge area below the shoulder.

E   The loss of sensation results from damage to the axillary nerve. On x-ray the humeral head lies anterior and inferior to the glenoid. The shoulder can be reduced with Kocher's manoeuvre. The elbow is flexed to 90° and traction applied. The arm is slowly externally rotated to about 90°, brought across the chest and then finally internally rotated.

A 40-year-old woman presents after a fall on an outstretched hand, with pain in the upper arm and a wrist drop.

K   The radial nerve is susceptible to injury with fracture of the humeral shaft as it winds around the humerus in the spiral groove.

40 Shoulder conditions

ANSWERS: 1G, 2E, 3A, 4K, 5D

A 21-year-old woman presents with a very painful shoulder locked in adduction and internal rotation following an epileptic fit.

G   Posterior dislocation is extremely rare but should always be considered in the epileptic patient with a painful shoulder post-seizure. On examination the coracoid process may be prominent and the humeral head felt posteriorly. The arm is held in the adducted, internally rotated position. A lateral film is essential to spot the posterior subluxation.

A 55-year-old man complains of shoulder pain aggravated in abduction of the arm between 60° and 120°.

E   This patient is describing a painful arc syndrome. The pain of supraspinatus tendonitis can be elicited if the examiner elevates an internally rotated arm causing the supraspinatus tendon to impinge against the anterior inferior acromion. This pain is reduced/alleviated if the test is repeated after injecting local anaesthetic into the subacromial space. Treatment includes the use of physiotherapy and patient education with respect to particular arm movements/activities. Corticosteroid/local anaesthetic injections are useful in the acute setting. Surgery is often necessary to arthroscopically increase the space for the tendon to move.

A 30-year-old bodybuilder presents with a painful shoulder after weightlifting. Flexing his elbow reveals a prominent lump in the upper arm.

A   This injury occurs after lifting/pulling activity. Good function usually returns without the need for surgery.

A 50-year-old man complains of a 9-month history of stiffness in the shoulder. The shoulder was originally extremely painful but now only the stiffness remains.

K   Adhesive capsulitis is more commonly known as 'frozen shoulder'. Examination should reveal marked reduction in passive and active movement. There may be some history of previous injury reported but this is not always present. There is no definitive treatment, but NSAIDs, intra-articular steroids and physiotherapy can reduce pain and increase range of movement in some patients.

A 65-year-old woman presents with shoulder pain and restricted movement in all directions. X-ray shows reduced joint space and subchondral sclerosis.

D   Reduced joint space, subchondral sclerosis, subchondral cysts and osteophytes are radiological features suggestive of osteoarthritis.

41 Knee conditions

ANSWERS: 1F, 2J, 3A, 4L, 5E

A 22-year-old figure-skater presents with a painful locked knee with limited extension following a twisting injury.

F   Meniscal tears usually result from a twisting injury. The displaced torn portion can become jammed between femur and tibia, resulting in locking. The medial meniscus is closely associated with the medial collateral ligament, so it is important to look out for dual pathology.

A 24-year-old footballer presents with a painful knee after landing awkwardly and twisting his knee after a header. With the quadriceps relaxed, there is excessive anterior glide of the tibia on the femur.

J   With the knee flexed at 90°, anterior glide of the tibia on the femur should only be about 0.5 cm. Excessive glide anteriorly implies anterior cruciate ligament damage; excessive glide posteriorly implies posterior cruciate ligament damage.

A 14-year-old girl successfully treated for rickets 3 years ago shows bow-legged deformity.

A   In valgus deformity the distal part is lateral to the midline.

A 16-year-old boy complains of a painful knee during exercise and a tender lump over the tibial tuberosity.

L   Osgood–Schlatter disease is more common in older children. Pain is felt particularly on direct palpation of the tibial tuberosity and when straight leg raising against resistance. The presence of a lump over the tibial tuberosity is diagnostic. Spontaneous recovery is usual but it is advisable to reduce sporting activity during this time.

A 50-year-old carpet layer presents with a swelling directly over the patella. The joint feels stable and there is no effusion.

E   Prepatellar bursitis was previously known as 'housemaid's knee'. The condition is usually treated by the use of firm bandaging and by abstaining from the kneeling position that has caused the injury.

42 Management of painful joints

ANSWERS: 1A, 2H, 3B, 4C, 5G

A 24-year-old man presented with lower back pain and stiffness that was worse in the morning. He has developed a thoracic kyphosis and has a hyperextended neck.

A   This is a presentation of ankylosing spondylitis. The thoracic kyphosis and hyperextension of the neck gives rise to the classical question-mark posture. Patients often report improvement of stiffness with hydrotherapy. Exercise is preferred to rest for the improvement of back symptoms.

An 80-year-old man with a 30-year history of rheumatoid arthritis presents to A&E with fever and pain in the right knee. On examination his right knee is red, hot and swollen. Aspirated synovial fluid is frankly purulent.

H   Aspiration of the joint and culture is required to establish whether the acutely swollen knee has resulted from inflammation, infection or a crystal arthropathy etc. Intravenous flucloxacillin plus benzylpenicillin is a popular broad-spectrum drug combination that is used until sensitivities are known. Surgery is required to wash out the knee.

A 65-year-old woman recently diagnosed with osteoarthritis requires medication for night pain.

B   Paracetamol should be prescribed before NSAIDs for relief of osteoarthritic pain. The use of NSAIDs for analgesia can be problematic in a chronic condition like osteoarthritis due to the risk of gastrointestinal bleeding with long-term use. This may be counteracted to some extent with concomitant use of proton pump inhibitors and prostaglandin analogues.

A 64-year-old woman who has been successfully treated for acute gout requires prophylactic medication.

C   Colchicine is an alternative to NSAIDs in an acute presentation of gout in patients in whom NSAIDs are contraindicated (e.g. allergy, heart failure). Allopurinol is a xanthine oxidase inhibitor which decreases the production of uric acid and is used only for prophylaxis. It should not be used in treatment of acute gout and in fact its use may actually provoke acute gout during that period.

A 65-year-old woman with painful shoulders due to polymyalgia rheumatica.

G   Oral prednisolone is the treatment of choice for polymyalgia rheumatica.

43 Foot conditions

ANSWERS: 1F, 2D, 3B, 4H

A 32-year-old marathon runner presents with persistent pain over the dorsum of the foot on weight-bearing.

F   A march fracture is the term used to describe a metatarsal stress fracture of the foot caused by excessive repetitive injury. It is therefore more common in athletes. Treatment is rest (an air-cast boot can be provided to reduce weight-bearing over the fracture site). Stress fractures are not always evident on plain radiographs, so the diagnosis may often be based on clinical examination alone for the first 2–3 weeks. MRI scans and bone scans are very helpful.

A 62-year-old man presents with persistent pain over the left big toe. On examination there is swelling and decreased range of movement over the first metatarsophalangeal joint.

D   Hallux rigidus is caused by arthritis at the metatarsophalangeal joint. The joint may be fused (arthrodesis) to treat the pain or an excision arthroplasty of the proximal half of the proximal phalynx (Keller's operation) may be performed. There are ongoing trials of joint replacements for this condition.

A 24-year-old man presents with pain in his right heel that is worse in the morning. On examination there is pain on passive dorsiflexion of the toes and when walking on tip-toes.

B   Plantar fasciitis is most common amongst runners, leading to the suggestion that it is a repetitive injury syndrome with microtrauma to the plantar fascia. However, there are also associations with inflammatory conditions (e.g. ankylosing spondylitis).

The plantar fascia arises from the medial tubercle of the calcaneus and fans out to insert on to the proximal phalanges and flexor tendon sheaths. On examination there may be tenderness over the anteromedial aspect of the heel (site of insertion) and on placing the flexor tendons under tension by passive dorsiflexion. Patients typically report pain in the morning which improves with ambulation but then worsens as activity increases. Conservative measures include reduction of precipitating exercise and use of arch supports as well as stretching and night splints. More invasive therapy (e.g. corticosteroid injections) is of unproven long-term benefit.

A 50-year-old woman complains of pain over the dorsal aspect of the PIP joint of the second toe. On examination there is a flexion deformity of the PIP with hyperextension at the DIP joint.

H   A hammer toe involves flexion of the proximal interphalangeal joint (PIP) and extension at the metatarsophalangeal joint and distal interphalangeal joint (DIP). Indication for surgery is failure of conservative measures (e.g. strapping to control pain). There are a number of options including arthrodesis of the PIP joint and flexor/extensor tenotomy.

44 Lower limb nerve lesion

ANSWERS: 1B, 2J, 3E, 4A

A 22-year-old footballer complains of weakness of dorsiflexion of the right foot after suffering an injury to the side of the knee.

B   The common peroneal nerve is susceptible to injury as it winds around the neck of the fibula. Injury results in foot drop (weakness of dorsiflexion and eversion). Sensation loss affects the area of skin over the anterolateral lower leg stretching to the dorsum of the foot (except for an area on the lateral side of the foot supplied by the sural nerve).

A 75-year-old patient presents with a profound foot drop several days after a hip hemiarthroplasty for a fractured neck of femur.

J   The sciatic nerve is at risk of injury during the posterior approach to the hip joint. Injury results in a profound foot drop with loss of all movement below the knee and paralysis of hamstrings.

A 38-year-old woman complains of sensation loss over the antero-medial aspect of the lower leg following varicose vein surgery.

E   The saphenous nerve arises from the posterior division of the femoral nerve and lies in close proximity to the long saphenous vein. It is therefore at risk of injury during long saphenous vein stripping surgery. It provides sensation to the anteromedial lower leg.

A 36-year-old man is brought to A&E after suffering penetrating trauma to the right popliteal fossa. On examination there is loss of active plantar flexion and loss of sensation over the sole of the foot.

A   The tibial nerve arises from the sciatic nerve just above the apex of the popliteal fossa. It passes in the midline of the popliteal fossa superficial to the popliteal vein and artery. It supplies sensation to the sole of the foot and motor supply to the flexors of the foot.

45 Upper limb nerve injury (i)

ANSWERS: 1B, 2C, 3I, 4F

A 25-year-old man complains of anaesthesia over a patch on his outer upper arm following anterior dislocation of the shoulder.

B   The axillary nerve is related to the medial aspect of the surgical neck of the humerus and is at risk of injury following fracture at this level or anterior dislocation of the shoulder. It is important to check the integrity of the nerve after anterior dislocation of the shoulder and to re-check the nerve status after reduction. It provides motor branches to the deltoid muscle and teres minor.

A 63-year-old man is found to have weakness of thumb abduction following carpal tunnel release surgery.

C   The median nerve motor supply to the small muscles of the hand can be remembered by the mnemonic LOAF (lateral two lumbricals, opponens pollicis, abductor pollicis brevis, and flexor pollicis brevis). The recurrent motor branch of the median nerve is at risk of injury during carpal tunnel surgery.

A young child presents to the orthopaedic clinic with claw hand and wasting of the small muscles of the hand. There is sensory deficit to light touch along the inner and upper forearm. The only medical history of note is that the child was delivered in the breech position.

I   This is a presentation of Klumpke's palsy which has resulted from upward traction on the arm during breech delivery causing injury to T1. Traction to the sympathetic chain can also give rise to an ipsilateral Horner's syndrome. Clawing results from the unopposed action of the long flexors.

A 7-year-old is found to have numbness over the medial one and a half fingers after suffering a supracondylar fracture of the humerus.

F   Injury of the ulnar nerve at the wrist gives rise to a distinctive claw hand. This is because paralysis of the lumbricals provides hyperextension of the metacarpals and paralysis of the interossei leads to flexion at the interphalangeal joints. Sensory deficit affects the little finger and medial half of the ring finger. Paradoxically a higher lesion at the level of the elbow, in this scenario, causes less clawing of the hand due to paralysis of the ulnar half of flexor digitorum profundus (unopposed flexion causes the clawing).

46 Upper limb nerve injury (ii)

ANSWERS: 1K, 2E, 3J

A 35-year-old patient is brought to A&E following a road traffic accident. She has suffered multiple fractures to the humerus and forearm bones. On examination there is an obvious wrist drop, loss of elbow extension and sensation loss over the first dorsal web space.

K   Clinical examination is useful to reveal the level of radial nerve injury. An injury at the level of the axilla is associated with loss of elbow extension along with the wrist drop and radial nerve sensory loss over the first dorsal web space.

With an injury at the level of the humerus shaft, elbow extension is preserved. An injury at the level of the wrist is associated with weakness in finger/wrist extension, but there is minimal wrist drop as the posterior interosseous nerve providing motor supply branches off above the level of the wrist.

A 45-year-old patient is brought to A&E after being assaulted. There is significant bruising over the right upper limb. On examination there is loss of forearm pronation and the hand is noted to deviate to the ulnar side when flexing the wrist.

E   Median nerve injury at the level of the elbow is associated with motor loss of the forearm pronators, and weakness of the forearm flexors and muscles of the thenar eminence. Sensation loss occurs over the radial three and a half fingers. An injury at wrist level spares the long flexors and sensation over the palmar aspect of the thenar eminence is spared (palmar cutaneous branch given off above wrist level).

A 30-year-old rugby player presents with winging of the scapula after suffering a blow to the ribs underneath an outstretched arm.

J   The long thoracic nerve supplies the serratus anterior which allows protraction of the shoulder. It is particularly at risk during breast/axillary surgery. The winging of the scapula deformity is best exemplified when the patient is pushing against a wall.

SECTION 3: VASCULAR SURGERY

QUESTIONS

47 Management of abdominal aortic aneurysm (AAA)

A	elective infrarenal endovascular stenting	F	femoropopliteal bypass graft
B	open aortoaortic repair	G	PET scan
C	open aortobiiliac repair	H	magnetic resonance imaging
D	ultrasound scan	I	sodium nitroprusside and propranolol
E	abdominal contrast CT scan	J	endoscopy

For each clinical scenario below, suggest the most appropriate management. Each option may be used only once.

1   A 75-year-old male with a long history of lumbar spinal and hip arthritis presents with sudden severe back pain, BP 100/50 mmHg, pulse 105/min.

2   An 82-year-old is found to have an uncomplicated 7.5 cm AAA on ultrasound as an incidental finding. He has had a previous emergency Hartmann's procedure for septic peritonitis secondary to benign diverticular perforation, 5 years earlier.

3   A 64-year-old man presents with an asymptomatic juxtarenal AAA measuring 6.5 cm in diameter. The left and right common iliac arteries measure 1.5 cm and 3.5 cm respectively. He has no other past medical history.

4   A 78-year-old woman presents 3 years after elective aortic aneurysm repair with a microcytic anaemia of unknown origin.

5   A 70-year-old male presents with a 1-week history of mid-back pain and right leg claudication at 150 yards. Imaging shows an enlarged dual lumen descending thoracic and abdominal aorta. He is known to be hypertensive.

Answers: see page 112

48 Treatment of peripheral vascular disease

A	heparin i.v.	G	Fogarty catheter
B	femoropopliteal bypass	H	percutaneous transluminal
C	conservative management		angioplasty
D	sympathectomy	I	aortobifemoral bypass
E	femorofemoral crossover graft	J	above-knee amputation
F	thrombolysis	K	below-knee amputation

For each clinical scenario below, suggest the most appropriate management.
Each option may be used only once.

1   A 75-year-old smoker presents with severe rest pain in her right leg. On examination there is advanced gangrene and cellulitis of the right foot with absent distal pulses. Angiography shows occluded crural vessels to the ankle.

2   A 73-year-old overweight smoker presents with pain in his legs after walking half a mile, which is relieved immediately by rest. Ankle brachial pressure index is 0.8.

3   A 62-year-old man presents with severe bilateral pain in the legs. He is known to suffer from impotence and buttock claudication. Femoral pulses are weak. Arteriography shows long occlusions on both common iliac arteries with good distal run-off. Angioplasty, though initially promising, proved unsuccessful.

4   A 65-year-old man complains of left calf claudication at 50 m. Angiography reveals a 10 cm stenosis of the superficial femoral artery.

5   A 74-year-old man with atrial fibrillation who suffered a stroke a week ago presents with an ischaemic cold foot. Duplex ultrasonography reveals acute occlusion of the popliteal artery.

Answers: see page 113

49 Complications of vascular surgery

A	acute mesenteric ischaemia	G	compartment syndrome
B	saphena varix	H	retroperitoneal haematoma
C	graft infection	I	sciatic nerve injury
D	endoleak	J	acute ischaemic cerebrovascular
E	trash foot		accident
F	vascular hernia	K	artery of Adamkiewicz injury

For each clinical scenario below, identify the most common complication. Each option may be used only once.

1   A 72-year-old underwent aortic aneurysm stent grafting 18 months earlier for a 5.8 cm AAA. The abdominal aorta remains asymptomatic but now measures 6.3 cm.

2   A 64-year-old man is unable to dorsiflex his right foot 24 hours after revascularization of acutely ischaemic foot on that side.

3   A 72-year-old woman presents with an erythematous tender groin lump which suddenly appeared 3 years after aortofemoral bypass.

4   A 65-year-old man presents with loss of power in both legs after aortic aneurysm repair.

5   A 57-year-old man is referred by the cardiologists with cool distal peripheries following repeated transfemoral catheterization of coronary arteries in the presence of aortic aneurysm.

Answers: see page 114

50 Treatment of peripheral arterial disease

A	carotid–carotid bypass	F	carotid artery stenting
B	carotid endarterectomy	G	warfarin
C	axillofemoral bypass	H	intravenous heparin
D	antiplatelet agent: statin	I	subclavian artery angioplasty
E	watch and wait	J	streptokinase

For each clinical scenario below, identify the most appropriate treatment. Each option may be used only once.

1 A 75-year-old patient with significant coronary artery disease presents with symptomatic restenosis of the right internal carotid artery. The anaesthetist feels that he is high risk for further surgery.

2 A 68-year-old man who initially presented to the physicians with amaurosis fugax is found to have 82 per cent left internal carotid artery stenosis.

3 A 58-year-old patient is found to have 50 per cent internal carotid artery stenosis. He is asymptomatic.

4 A 65-year-old woman has recently taken up tennis to stay fit. She reports episodes of syncope during play.

Answers: see page 116

ANSWERS

47 Management of abdominal aortic aneurysm

ANSWERS: 1E, 2A, 3C, 4J, 5I

A 75-year-old male with a long history of lumbar spinal and hip arthritis presents with sudden severe back pain, BP 100/50 mmHg, pulse 105/min.

E   Abdominal aortic aneurysms are asymptomatic in most patients and often found incidentally. Sudden-onset severe back pain could prove an important early warning of an impending potentially catastrophic complication especially if new or different. Tachycardia and hypotension may suggest a contained leak. Emergency intravenous contrast CT is the investigation of choice in this setting.

An 82-year-old is found to have an uncomplicated 7.5 cm AAA on ultrasound as an incidental finding. He has had a previous emergency Hartmann's procedure for septic peritonitis secondary to benign diverticular perforation, 5 years earlier.

A   Surgery is recommended for aortic aneurysms greater than 5.5 cm diameter. This may be performed using the open or endovascular technique. The latter is associated with lower perioperative morbidity and mortality and may be preferable in elderly patients with significant systemic comorbidity and for the potentially hostile abdomen.

A 64-year-old man presents with an asymptomatic juxtarenal AAA measuring 6.5 cm in diameter. The left and right common iliac arteries measure 1.5 cm and 3.5 cm respectively. He has no other past medical history.

C   Simple infrarenal endovascular stenting is contraindicated in juxtarenal aneurysms due to lack of an appropriate proximal landing segment of non-aneurysmal aorta below the renal arteries. Although there may be a role for fenestrated stenting, open repair is probably more appropriate in the younger patient with unsuitable endovascular anatomy.

A 78-year-old woman presents 3 years after elective aortic aneurysm repair with a microcytic anaemia of unknown origin.

J   Aortoenteric fistula (AEF) is an uncommon, often late complication of open repair and may present as unexplained anaemia. AEF is an uncommon catastrophic communication between the aorta and the gastrointestinal tract. Primary AEF is very rare with < 200 reported cases. Secondary AEF is a more common late complication of open AAA repairs (about 1 per cent). The overlying duodenum is involved in

80 per cent of cases. The initial 'herald bleed' presenting as melaena or haematochezia with minimal haemodynamic consequence, is followed hours or days later by a catastrophic gastrointestinal bleed. A high index of suspicion is vital.

Endoscopy is the procedure of choice and is diagnostic in 90 per cent of cases. CT, MRI and transluminal angiography may also be useful. Surgery is mandatory and associated with 60–90 per cent mortality, compared to 100 per cent if untreated.

A 70-year-old male presents with a 1-week history of mid-back pain and right leg claudication at 150 yards. Imaging shows an enlarged dual lumen descending thoracic and abdominal aorta. He is known to be hypertensive.

I   Aortic dissection (AD) is more common than aortic rupture and, if untreated, mortality increases by 1 per cent every hour for the first 48 hours. Type A dissection involves the ascending aorta and aortic arch. Type B originates in the descending thoracic or thoracoabdominal aorta and may involve the arch but not the ascending aorta. AD may present with tearing, acute midsternal chest pain (ascending) or interscapular back pain (descending). Propagation may present as migratory pain and peripheral and visceral ischaemia as branches are involved.

CT and increasingly MR angiography is the investigation of choice. Transoesophageal echocardiography is a reliable second choice. Emergency surgery is indicated for acute type A dissection. Uncomplicated type B dissection is best managed medically with rapid control of blood pressure using sodium nitroprusside and beta-blockers (e.g. labetalol).

48 Treatment of peripheral vascular disease

ANSWERS: 1K, 2C, 3I, 4H, 5G

A 75-year-old smoker presents with severe rest pain in her right leg. On examination there is advanced gangrene and cellulitis of the right foot with absent distal pulses. Angiography shows occluded crural vessels to the ankle.

K   Angioplastic or surgical revascularization is unlikely to succeed where crural vessels are occluded below the ankle. It is especially important to adequately counsel the patient for such a measure. Forefoot amputation will not be advisable in a non-revascularized foot. A below-knee amputation may represent the best option to avert the risk of systemic sepsis and restore quality of life.

A 73-year-old overweight smoker presents with pain in his legs after walking half a mile, which is relieved immediately by rest. Ankle brachial pressure index is 0.8.

C   Claudication distance (distance travelled before he gets pain) of 500 yards may be considered reasonable for this patient, obviating invasive treatment in the first instance. Ankle brachial pressure index of above 0.9 is normal. Patients with claudication but no rest pain usually have a value that is between 0.6 and 0.9. A value below 0.6 is associated with rest pain and critical ischaemia. Conservative management consists of stopping smoking, taking up physical exercising such as walking and weight reduction. Medical intervention includes the treatment of diabetes, hypertension and hyperlipidaemia. Daily low-dose aspirin is indicated.

A 62-year-old man presents with severe bilateral pain in the legs. He is known to suffer from impotence and buttock claudication. Femoral pulses are weak. Arteriography shows long occlusions on both common iliac arteries with good distal run-off. Angioplasty, though initially promising, proved unsuccessful.

I   The distal aorta bifurcates into the two common iliac arteries (median sacral branch is also given off). The common iliac artery divides to form the external and internal iliac arteries. The external iliac artery passes under the inguinal ligament to become the femoral artery. Angioplasty and stenting of the iliac arteries is the first option and is successful in most cases. Otherwise, as in this case, an aortobifemoral bypass should restore appropriate axial flow to both legs.

A 65-year-old man complains of left calf claudication at 50 m. Angiography reveals a 10 cm stenosis of the superficial femoral artery.

H   The superficial femoral artery becomes the popliteal artery in the popliteal fossa. Percutaneous transluminal angioplasty is the treatment of choice for this scenario where there is significant stenotic or occlusive disease of the superficial femoral artery.

A 74-year-old man with atrial fibrillation who suffered a stroke a week ago presents with an ischaemic cold foot. Duplex ultrasonography reveals acute occlusion of the popliteal artery.

G   With acute ischaemia secondary to embolism, surgical embolectomy with a Fogarty catheter is indicated. Intra-arterial local thrombolysis involves the use of thrombolytics like streptokinase/tissue plasminogen activator (t-PA). Thrombolysis would be contraindicated in this scenario due to his recent history of stroke.

49 Complications of vascular surgery

ANSWERS: 1D, 2G, 3C, 4K, 5E

A 72-year-old underwent aortic aneurysm stent grafting 18 months earlier for a 5.8 cm AAA. The abdominal aorta remains asymptomatic but now measures 6.3 cm.

D   Endoleak is a common complication of endovascular aneurysm repair
         representing a failure of the stent to exclude a weakened aneurysm
         sac from the systemic circulation. The presence of an endoleak with
         increasing sac volume suggests continuing pressurization of the sac.
         The risk of catastrophic rupture remains. Treatment can in most cases
         be accomplished endovascularly.

         **A 64-year-old man is unable to dorsiflex his right foot 24 hours after
         revascularization of acutely ischaemic foot on that side.**

G   Ischaemic reperfusion following revascularization of a prolonged acutely
         ischaemic limb may result in a significantly increased compartment
         pressure. Compartment syndrome is limb-threatening and occurs when
         perfusion pressure drops below tissue pressure in a confined anatomical
         space. Consequently, perfusion and tissue oxygenation cease as the
         contents of the compartment become increasingly ischaemic. The
         limb is swollen, tender and painful at rest or with passive movement
         progressing to loss of sensation, paraesthesia and paralysis. Fasciotomy
         is both prophylactic and therapeutic. The former is advisable following
         prolonged severe ischaemia.

         **A 72-year-old woman presents with an erythematous tender groin
         lump which suddenly appeared 3 years after aortofemoral bypass.**

C   Low-virulence prosthetic graft infection may present many years after
         the initial operative procedure. A recent review reported an incidence
         of 7 per cent vascular graft infection in 410 patients (*Vasc Endov
         Surg* 2005;39:115). Misdiagnosis as a strangulated groin hernia may
         present the surgeon with an unpleasant surprise for which he may be
         unprepared.

         **A 65-year-old man presents with loss of power in both legs after
         aortic aneurysm repair.**

K   Spinal cord ischaemic paralysis is an uncommon but well-recognized
         complication of aortic surgery, especially the distal thoracic segment.
         This complication is often attributed to the loss of the artery of
         Adamkiewicz, a branch of the thoracic aorta supplying the distal
         two-thirds of the spinal cord via the anterior spinal artery.

         **A 57-year-old man is referred by the cardiologists with cool distal
         peripheries following repeated transfemoral catheterization of coro-
         nary arteries in the presence of aortic aneurysm.**

E   Repeated instrumentation of aneurysmal vessels may result in distal
         embolization of sac thrombi and intra-arterial debris presenting with
         foot ischaemia that is known as 'trash foot'. The diagnosis is often
         clinically obvious with the unwelcome combination of patent proximal
         pulses and acutely ischaemic foot following open or percutaneous
         intervention. It is a disconcerting complication associated with

significant risk of limb loss. Prevention and treatment includes heparin, embolectomy, lumbar sympathectomy, aspirin, Rheomacrodex and prostaglandins. Rest pain and tissue loss may necessitate amputation.

50 Treatment of peripheral arterial disease

ANSWERS: 1F, 2B, 3D, 4I

A 75-year-old patient with significant coronary artery disease presents with symptomatic restenosis of the right internal carotid artery. The anaesthetist feels that he is high risk for further surgery.

F   Carotid angioplasty and stenting is a viable, rapidly growing alternative to surgery especially in clinical scenarios where surgery is considered high risk (e.g. symptomatic restenosis, high carotid bifurcation, post-irradiation, previous neck surgery with contralateral nerve injury, and synchronous coronary carotid disease).

A 68-year-old man who initially presented to the physicians with amaurosis fugax is found to have 82 per cent left internal carotid artery stenosis.

B   Carotid endarterectomy is clearly superior to medical therapy alone in symptomatic patients with > 70 per cent internal carotid stenosis (9 per cent vs 26 per cent 2-year stroke rate; North American Symptomatic Carotid Endarterectomy Trial (NASCET), European Carotid Surgery Trial (ECST)). Surgery is only marginally beneficial in symptomatic patients with moderate stenosis (50–69 per cent), especially in men. The recent UK Asymptomatic Carotid Surgery Trial (ACST) has also shown benefit for surgery in asymptomatic patients with severe stenosis, reducing the 5-year stroke risk by 50 per cent. Surgery is not beneficial in patients with asymptomatic mild to moderate stenosis, occluded carotid, severe neurological deficit following a stroke, and severe continuing life-limiting medical illness.

A 58-year-old patient is found to have 50 per cent internal carotid artery stenosis. He is asymptomatic.

D   Cerebrovascular accident (stroke) is the third leading cause of death in the UK. Eighty per cent of strokes are ischaemic, and of these 80 per cent are related to the carotid artery distribution. Atherosclerotic disease is responsible for more than 90 per cent of carotid ischaemic events. Treatment options are medical, surgical and endovascular. All stand to benefit from cardiovascular risk reduction with antiplatelet agents (aspirin, clopidogrel), statins, weight reduction, control of hypertension and diabetes, smoking cessation and active lifestyle.

A 65-year-old woman has recently taken up tennis to stay fit. She reports episodes of syncope during play.

I   Subclavian steal syndrome occurs when, as a result of proximal
         subclavian or brachiocephalic artery occlusion, there is retrograde
         diverted flow, via the vertebral artery to the distal subclavian, causing
         cerebral or brainstem ischaemia. The patients are usually asymptomatic
         until increased upper limb muscular activity makes a greater demand
         (steal) on the brain circulation causing transient ischaemia, often
         presenting as vertigo or syncope. Absence of a pulse and differential
         upper limb hypotension add to the diagnosis which can be confirmed
         on duplex ultrasound, and transluminal CT or MR angiography. The
         occluded subclavian origin may be revascularized by angioplasty/
         stenting or surgical bypass.

SECTION 4: UROLOGY

QUESTIONS

51 Haematuria

A	Wilms' tumour	F	polycystic kidney disease
B	neuroblastoma	G	adrenal carcinoma
C	renal cell carcinoma (RCC)	H	rhabdomyolysis
D	fibroepithelial polyp	I	renal calculus
E	squamous cell carcinoma of the bladder	J	transitional cell carcinoma

For each clinical scenario below, suggest the most likely cause for the haematuria. Each option may be used only once.

1 A 75-year-old woman has had a UTI treated but has persistent microscopic haematuria seen on urine dipstick. She's not worried but her GP refers her to the one-stop haematuria clinic.

2 A 50-year-old man with weight loss, loss of appetite and shortness of breath has recently noticed a left-sided varicocoele which does not disappear on lying supine.

3 A 35-year-old man with new-onset hypertension is admitted to hospital for investigation. His creatinine is 134 mmol/L. After imaging he is advised to tell his brother to undergo family screening and genetic counselling.

4 An 18-year-old is travelling in the Australian outback during his gap year. He returns to London to run the marathon which he does successfully. The next day he attends A&E concerned about his dark red urine. He is otherwise completely asymptomatic but is admitted to hospital.

5 A 29-year-old man from Egypt presents with weight loss and haematuria. Pseudotubercles and nodules seen on cystoscopy are biopsied.

ANSWERS: see page 128

52 Testicular conditions

A	varicocoele	F	seminoma
B	chronic orchitis	G	epididymal cyst
C	ectopic testis	H	indirect inguinal hernia
D	hydrocoele	I	acute epididymo-orchitis
E	non-seminomatous testicular cancer	J	testicular atrophy
		K	testicular torsion

For each clinical scenario below, suggest the most likely diagnosis. Each option may be used only once.

1 A 52-year-old man presents with a testicular swelling that has increased in size gradually over a period of years. On examination the swelling transilluminates and the testis cannot be felt separate from the swelling.

2 A 40-year-old man complains of severe pain and swelling over the last 48 hours in his right scrotum. Testis and epididymis are very tender. He reports that he has had unprotected intercourse recently.

3 A 20-year-old man with a history of undescended testes presents with weight loss and a hard painless testicular lump.

4 A 9-year-old boy wakes at night crying from severe pain in the testis associated with vomiting.

5 A 45-year-old man presents with a left-sided fluctuant scrotal swelling. On standing the swelling worsens.

ANSWERS: see page 130

53 Bladder outlet obstruction

A	phimosis	F	clot retention
B	urethral stricture	G	pelvic mass
C	pregnancy	H	bladder stones
D	prostate cancer	I	urethral diverticula
E	benign prostatic hypertrophy (BPH)	J	urethral tumour
		K	bladder tumour

For each clinical scenario below, suggest the most likely cause for bladder outlet obstruction. Each option may be used only once.

1   A 75-year-old man describes difficulty passing urine associated with a noticeable white scar and ballooning of his foreskin.

2   A 58-year-old woman is due to undergo hysterectomy. She has chronic renal failure.

3   A 35-year-old man complains of difficulty passing urine. He has a history of multiple hospital admissions as a child for recurrent urine infections. He had bilateral vesico-ureteric reflux for which he required repeated catheterization.

4   A 63-year-old man 1 week post-transurethral resection of the prostate (TURP) underwent a successful trial without catheter 2 days ago and was discharged. He reattends in severe discomfort, being no longer able to pass urine.

5   An 84-year-old man complains of difficulty passing urine, nocturia, hesitancy and terminal dribbling. His prostate-specific antigen (PSA) is normal for his age.

Answers: see page 131

54 Management of prostate cancer

A	radical prostatectomy	G	anti-androgen medication
B	bilateral orchidectomy	H	luteinizing hormone releasing
C	transurethral resection of		hormone analogue
	prostate	I	long-term catheter and hospice
D	watch and wait	J	family screening
E	radiotherapy	K	repeat PSA
F	bone scan and dexamethasone		

For each clinical scenario below, suggest the most likely course of management. Each option may be used only once.

1   A 64-year-old man with a history of hesitancy, nocturia, frequency and terminal dribbling fails a trial without catheter despite being on an alpha-blocker. Rectal examination reveals a smooth enlarged prostate. He is otherwise fit and healthy and his biopsy results are negative for cancer.

2   A 66-year-old man has recently had a routine blood screen and is reported to have an elevated PSA of 5.5 ng/mL. He is otherwise asymptomatic.

3   A 34-year-old man attends your clinic reporting that his twin brother has been diagnosed with prostate cancer.

4   A 73-year-old man with prostate cancer attends your clinic complaining of new-onset back pain.

5   A 52-year-old man is diagnosed with prostate cancer and staging confirms the absence of secondary spread of disease.

Answers: see page 133

55 Urinary incontinence (diagnosis/management)

A mid-stream urine microscopy, culture and sensitivity (MCS)
B cystoscopy
C flow rate
D ultrasound of kidneys and bladder residual
E video urodynamics
F DMSA scan
G intravenous urogram
H MAG3 scan
I urethrogram
J pelvic floor exercises
K bladder augmentation

For each clinical scenario below, suggest the most suitable investigation/management. Each option may be used only once.

1 A 35-year-old woman presents 2 years after the birth of her child with urinary leakage on coughing, standing and sneezing.

2 A 25-year-old man presents with slowing of his urinary flow and terminal urethral dribbling. He has a past history of a treated sexually transmitted disease.

3 A 75-year-old woman presents with recent onset of severe urinary urgency and bladder pain. Urinary dipstick shows no nitrates, protein 1+ and blood 2+.

4 An 80-year-old man presents to the urology clinic with poor flow, frequency and nocturia. He is noted to have an elevated creatinine.

5 A 40-year-old woman who has had two previous colposuspensions for urinary incontinence now complains of mixed urge and stress leakage.

Answers: see page 135

56 Management of renal stones

A	simple analgesia and discharge home with outpatient follow-up	F	percutaneous nephrolithotomy (PCNL)
B	emergency nephrectomy	G	embolization
C	MAG3 scan	H	nephrostomy
D	extracorporeal shock wave lithotripsy (ESWL)	I	ultrasound kidneys
E	ureteroscopy and laser fragmentation	J	intravenous antibiotics
		K	retrograde ureteric stenting

For each clinical scenario below, suggest the most appropriate management option. Each option may be used only once.

1 A 40-year-old man has had a PCNL to treat a renal 2.5 cm stone. At the end of the procedure there is gross bleeding from the nephrostomy track. Nephrostomy tamponade fails to stop the bleeding.

2 A 35-year-old woman, in the first trimester of pregnancy, presents with severe right loin pain.

3 A 50-year-old woman with diabetes presents with severe left loin pain, pyrexia, tachycardia and a white cell count of 24 000. Intravenous urogram shows no function on the initial 10-minute film.

4 A 37-year-old man presents with left renal colic. CT urogram shows a 5 mm stone in the lower third of the left ureter with moderate hydronephrosis.

5 A 27-year-old man presents with severe loin pain. Plain x-ray shows a staghorn calculus.

Answers: see page 137

57 Lumps in the groin

A	maldescended testis	G	varicocoele
B	femoral aneurysm	H	seminoma
C	hydrocoele	I	scrotal carcinoma
D	lipoma of the cord	J	saphena varix
E	inguinal hernia	K	inguinal lymphadenopathy
F	psoas abscess		

For each of the clinical scenarios below, give the most likely cause for the clinical findings. Each option may be used only once.

1   An incidental lump is found during inguinal hernia repair. It is benign and left alone.

2   A 60-year-old smoker complains of a throbbing lump in his right groin. Examination reveals an expansile pulsation in the mass.

3   A new significant groin lump is found in a 9-year-old boy who had previously undergone unsuccessful laparoscopy for undescended testis.

4   An 80-year-old man has been attending his GP for 3 years with an enlarging right-sided scrotal mass which disappears on lying flat but worsens during the day. The GP cannot get above the mass, nor does it transilluminate.

5   A 69-year-old woman with right leg pain is diagnosed with a deep vein thrombosis on Doppler investigation. On examination there are firm rubbery matted masses in both groins.

Answers: see page 138

58 Urological imaging/intervention

A	transurethral resection of the prostate	H	high-intensity frequency ultrasound (HIFU) prostate ablation
B	retrograde ureterogram		
C	nephrostomy	I	radical prostatectomy
D	micturating cystourethrogram	J	nephrocystourethrectomy and ileal conduit formation
E	ultrasound of urinary tract		
F	intravenous urogram (IVU)	K	active surveillance
G	furosemide		

For each clinical scenario below, suggest the most suitable next step. Each option may be used only once.

1   A 45-year-old man has muscle-invasive transitional cell carcinoma of the bladder extending to multiple sites along the right ureter and involving the renal pelvis.

2   An 83-year-old man with a PSA of 10 ng/mL and positive transrectal ultrasound (TRUS) guided biopsy results denies lower urinary tract symptoms. He does not want any surgical intervention.

3   A 45-year-old man has raised PSA of 29 ng/mL and positive TRUS biopsy results. His brother died of prostate cancer aged 60 years.

4   A 30-year-old man with a history of renal stones has been on a business trip and taken diclofenac and codeine throughout his meetings. He returns to attend A&E with further pain.

5   A 15-year-old female complains of severe loin pain when voiding.

Answers: see page 140

59 Renal masses/tumours

A	lymphoma	G	staghorn calculus
B	polycystic kidney	H	perirenal haematoma
C	simple cyst	I	squamous cell carcinoma
D	sarcoma	J	medullary sponge kidney
E	adrenal mass	K	renal cell carcinoma
F	renal abscess		

For each clinical scenario below, suggest the most likely cause for the renal mass. Each option may be used only once.

1   A 57-year-old man with acute cholecystitis undergoes ultrasound scanning of the abdomen. An incidental note of a renal lesion is made. The patient is informed and reassured that it is benign.

2   A 46-year-old woman presents with a 3-month history of haematuria, weight loss, fevers, lethargy and loin pain, and a palpable loin mass. She has no significant past medical history, or travel history.

3   A 23-year-old man attends A&E having fallen off a motorbike at 30 miles per hour. He presents with an expanding left loin mass, bruising and haematuria.

4   A 37-year-old HIV-positive male presents to the clinic with haematuria, swinging pyrexia and raised white cell count. On examination he has a tender left loin mass.

Answers: see page 141

ANSWERS

51 Haematuria

ANSWERS: 1J, 2C, 3F, 4H, 5E

A 75-year-old woman has had a UTI treated but has persistent
microscopic haematuria seen on urine dipstick. She's not worried but
her GP refers her to the one-stop haematuria clinic.

J   Painless haematuria is the presenting complaint in over 80 per cent
of patients with transitional cell carcinoma. Other symptoms include
frequency, dysuria, urgency, loin pain secondary to ureteric obstruction, recurrent urinary tract infections or microscopic haematuria.
Investigation involves urine cytology, intravenous urography, ultrasound scanning and flexible cystoscopy.

Risk factors include smoking, chronic ingestion of analgesics (e.g. phen-
acetin), cyclophosphamide therapy, and history of radiotherapy to the
pelvis. Workers in chemical industries involving exposure to aniline
dyes or aromatic hydrocarbons such as naphthylamine and benzidine
are also at risk.

Most bladder cancers are superficial at presentation and consequently
treatment involves cystoscopic resection (TURBT) with intravesical
chemotherapy. Other treatments include cystectomy, chemotherapy,
radiotherapy and immunotherapy with intravesical BCG.

A 50-year-old man with weight loss, loss of appetite and shortness
of breath has recently noticed a left-sided varicocoele which does not
disappear on lying supine.

C   The classic triad of haematuria, loin pain and a palpable abdominal
mass is found in fewer than 20 per cent of those presenting with renal
cell carcinoma. In EMQs, look out for a coexisting paraneoplastic syndrome such as anaemia, polycythaemia (due to excess erythropoeitin
secretion) or hypercalcaemia (due to PTH-related peptide secretion) that
can occur in up to a third of patients.

Contrast CT will show the macroscopic features of the RCC as well as
any further liver or lung 'cannonball' metastases. Solitary metastases
can be excised and long-term survival is not uncommon.

RCC and testicular teratomas show a propensity for the development
of solitary pulmonary metastases. Treatment in the absence of distant
metastases is by radical (open or laparoscopic) nephrectomy.

Five per cent of RCCs are associated with direct tumour extension
into the inferior vena cava (IVC), and possibly the right atrium, in
which case thrombectomy is also combined with the nephrectomy. The

infradiaphragmatic portion of the IVC can be approached by venotomy and repair. Supradiaphragmatic extension requires cardiopulmonary bypass for tumour removal.

A 35-year-old man with new-onset hypertension is admitted to hospital for investigation. His creatinine is 134 mmol/L. After imaging he is advised to tell his brother to undergo family screening and genetic counselling.

F   Polycystic kidney disease (PCKD) occurs via autosomal dominant inheritance usually presenting in the fourth decade with loin pain and/ or haematuria as a result of haemorrhage into a cyst. Other symptoms/ signs include abdominal discomfort due to local pressure effects, hypertension or symptoms of chronic renal failure.

Family members are routinely screened and are thus diagnosed at a pre-clinical stage by ultrasound imaging of the kidneys. Autosomal dominant PCKD is the most common inherited disorder leading to renal failure due to replacement of the substance of the kidney by cysts. Cysts may be found in the liver (30 per cent), spleen (15 per cent) and pancreas (10 per cent).

PCKD accounts for about 10 per cent of patients receiving renal replacement therapy, and a significant proportion of these will undergo renal transplantation.

An 18-year-old is travelling in the Australian outback during his gap year. He returns to London to run the marathon which he does successfully. The next day he attends A&E concerned about his dark red urine. He is otherwise completely asymptomatic but is admitted to hospital.

H   Rhabdomyolysis is a syndrome caused by injury to skeletal muscle. Causes include burns, trauma, alcohol abuse and drug abuse. In this case the trauma is long-distance running. The injury to skeletal muscle results in leakage of intracellular contents into the plasma and can ultimately cause acute renal failure, electrolyte disturbances, hyperkalaemia and arrhythmias.

Immediately after muscle injury, creatine kinase levels rise and ongoing muscle injury will result in continuing elevation. In addition, myoglobin is released into the urine which is responsible for the dark discoloration. Urinalysis may test positive for blood but negative for red blood cells. Mainstay of management involves aggressive fluid resuscitation and close monitoring of urine output. Urine alkalinization may be helpful to prevent acute tubular necrosis. Indications for dialysis include persistent metabolic acidosis, oliguric renal failure, persistent hyperkalaemia and pulmonary oedema.

A 29-year-old man from Egypt presents with weight loss and haematuria. Pseudotubercles and nodules seen on cystoscopy are biopsied.

E   Schistosomiasis (bilharzia) has affected dwellers of the Nile valley for centuries. The trematode penetrates the skin and flourishes in the liver. Eventually, a male and female pair make their way to the inferior mesenteric vein and reach the vesical venous plexus through the portosystemic anastomotic channels. The female lays ova in the bladder. Cystoscopic examination may reveal bilharzia pseudotubercles and bilharzia nodules and biopsies of scanty patches can confirm the diagnosis. Schistosomiasis of the bladder which has been neglected for years can result in squamous cell carcinoma as a result of metaplasia.

52 Testicular conditions

ANSWERS: 1D, 2I, 3E, 4K, 5A

A 52-year-old man presents with a testicular swelling that has increased in size gradually over a period of years. On examination the swelling transilluminates and the testis cannot be felt separate from the swelling.

D   A hydrocoele is a collection of fluid in the tunica vaginalis. As the fluid of the hydrocoele surrounds the body of the testis, the underlying testis is impalpable. Primary hydrocoele is idiopathic. Secondary hydrocoele occurs secondary to trauma, tumour and infection. Aspiration is discouraged unless malignancy has been ruled out. Surgical excision is by either Jaboulay's or Lord's procedure.

A 40-year-old man complains of severe pain and swelling over the last 48 hours in his right scrotum. Testis and epididymis are very tender. He reports that he has had unprotected intercourse recently.

I   The onset of symptoms here are more insidious in nature than in acute torsion. There may be signs of urinary tract infection (i.e. frequency and dysuria). *Chlamydia* and other sources of sexually transmitted infections are more common in younger men whereas bacteria such as *Escherichia coli* are more common in older men. Symptoms include dysuria, fever, throbbing constant pain and tender swollen epididymis. Antibiotic therapy is the treatment of choice. Occasionally surgical exploration may be necessary if there is doubt about the diagnosis.

A 20-year-old man with a history of undescended testes presents with weight loss and a hard painless testicular lump.

E   Seminomas are the more common of the germ cell tumours. They usually present between the age of 30 and 40 years, whereas non-seminomatous testicular cancers commonly present earlier (20–30 years). Undescended testes are an important risk factor for testicular tumours.

        The most common presentation is of a palpable scrotal mass/scrotal pain. Less common presentations include gynaecomastia, reduced libido and infertility (tumour secreting hormones).

Assessment includes chest x-ray to identify 'cannonball pulmonary metastases', tumour markers (alpha-fetoprotein (AFP) and beta-HCG used to monitor germ cell tumours), ultrasound and full staging CT once diagnosis is confirmed. Note that 40 per cent of seminomas classically do not produce AFP or β-HCG.

Inguinal-approach orchidectomy with early clamping of the spermatic cord vessels (preventing tumour dissemination during mobilization of the testis) is the surgical treatment of choice. The spermatic cord is ligated at the deep inguinal ring and the structures below are removed. Patients with evidence of extratesticular disease on CT staging receive chemoradiotherapy with good response.

A 9-year-old boy wakes at night crying from severe pain in the testis associated with vomiting.

K   There is a congenital anatomical abnormality that allows torsion of the whole testicle ('bell-clapper testes'). A normal testicle is fixed within the tunica vaginalis and cannot twist. The pain of torsion is severe and often associated with nausea and vomiting. Testicular torsion is a urological emergency and prompt surgical intervention (within 6 hours of onset of symptoms) is indicated to ensure salvage of the affected testis. Acute epididymo-orchitis can give a similar, albeit more insidious, presentation, but it is always best to explore surgically to rule out torsion if there is any doubt. It is important to remember that torsion of the testis can occur spontaneously without any history of trauma.

A 45-year-old man presents with a left-sided fluctuant scrotal swelling. On standing the swelling worsens.

A   Varicocoeles are classically described as a 'bag of worms' collection of dilated veins. Patients often complain of a dragging aching sensation in the scrotum. Varicocoele is associated with infertility and so operative intervention is recommended. This can be carried out by an abdominal or inguinal approach. Right-sided varicocele is unusual and requires investigation of the right kidney.

53 Bladder outlet obstruction

ANSWERS: 1A, 2G, 3B, 4F, 5E

A 75-year-old man describes difficulty passing urine associated with a noticeable white scar and ballooning of his foreskin.

A   Phimosis is a fibrous contraction of the preputial aperture which makes it impossible to retract the foreskin. The resulting ballooning of the foreskin and build-up of smegma leads to recurrent balanitis, as well as secondary bladder outlet obstruction. Treatment requires circumcision.

A 58-year-old woman is due to undergo hysterectomy. She has chronic renal failure.

G   In women of this age group, gynaecological surgery and cancers of pelvic organs are important causes of obstruction. With a delay in diagnosis, a chronic pressure in the pelvis results in chronic renal failure. Obstructive nephropathy should be considered especially in uraemic patients without a previous history of renal disease, hypertension or diabetes. In this case the patient has had a pelvic mass for which she requires surgery in order to prevent further renal damage. Causes include carcinoma of the colon/cervix/bladder/uterus, uterine fibroids and uterine leiomyomata.

A 35-year-old man complains of difficulty passing urine. He has a history of multiple hospital admissions as a child for recurrent urine infections. He had bilateral vesico-ureteric reflux for which he required repeated catheterization.

B   This is a classic example of the long-term sequelae of paediatric urological cases. Multiple hospital admissions with urinary tract infections can lead to long-term hospital stay with indwelling catheters. Repeated trauma can result in urethral stricture as an adult which requires surgical correction.

A 63-year-old man 1 week post-TURP underwent a successful trial without catheter 2 days ago and was discharged. He reattends in severe discomfort, being no longer able to pass urine.

F   Haematuria is a common cause of urinary retention. In this case the bladder outlet obstruction is a result of the urethra being blocked by a residual clot from the operation or from rebleeding. Patients with persistent postoperative bleeding require catheterization with three-way irrigation to prevent obstructing bladder outflow. The irrigation fluid is glycine. This is used to avoid TUR syndrome.

An 84-year-old man complains of difficulty passing urine, nocturia, hesitancy and terminal dribbling. His PSA is normal for his age.

E   In young and middle-aged men, renal calculi are the most common cause of at least temporary urinary obstruction. After the age of 60, urinary obstruction is most common in men secondary to prostatic hypertrophy; prostate cancer accounts for occasional cases. Symptoms of prostatism are poor flow, feeling of incomplete emptying and hesitancy. In addition, patients may or may not complain of frequency, urgency, dribbling, decrease in voiding stream, and the need to double void (pis-en-deux).

Urodynamic studies are useful. A flow-rate study with a voided volume of 200 mL or more can be used; Q_{max} (maximum urinary flow rate) of less than 10 mL/s indicates bladder outlet obstruction.

Ultrasound scan of the abdomen measures post-micturition residual bladder volume. A residual volume of more than 100 mL suggests chronic urinary retention. A transrectal ultrasound scan of the prostate confirms BPH and if a mass lesion is seen, fine needle aspiration for cytology or Tru-cut biopsy can be performed.

Significant BPH can be treated by transurethral resection of prostate. A resectoscope is inserted during cystoscopy and prostatic chippings sent for histological confirmation of diagnosis. Complications of the procedure include infection, haemorrhage, clot retention, urethral stricture, incontinence, retrograde ejaculation, impotence and transurethral syndrome. The latter syndrome is caused by excessive absorption of glycine irrigation fluid. The resultant fluid overload and hyponatraemia manifests as hypotension, bradycardia, confusion, nausea and, in severe cases, convulsions.

Treatment involves infusion of 2 M saline solution combined with furosemide.

54 Management of prostate cancer

ANSWERS: 1C, 2K, 3J, 4F, 5A

A 64-year-old man with a history of hesitancy, nocturia, frequency and terminal dribbling fails a trial without catheter despite being on an alpha-blocker. Rectal examination reveals a smooth enlarged prostate. He is otherwise fit and healthy and his biopsy results are negative for cancer.

C   The cardinal symptoms of benign prostatic hypertrophy are poor flow, a feeling of incomplete emptying and hesitancy. Other symptoms may be as described in this question (frequency, nocturia and terminal dribbling). These patients can develop urinary retention and present to A&E requiring catheterization. They are started on an alpha-receptor antagonist which relaxes the bladder neck and a trial without catheter can be attempted. Long-term urinary retention can lead to chronic renal failure, which manifests as uraemic symptoms and an elevated serum creatinine level. This patient has had a transrectal ultrasound scan and biopsy to confirm it is benign enlargement. There are no contraindications to surgery so he can undergo transurethral resection of prostate. If he did have cancer then he could be offered radical prostatectomy.

A 66-year-old man has recently had a routine blood screen and is reported to have an elevated PSA of 5.5 ng/mL. He is otherwise asymptomatic.

K   An elevated PSA can occur for multiple reasons such as urinary tract infection, trauma and catheterization. An incidental finding of an elevated PSA must therefore be repeated to check the result. If it remains elevated, despite being asymptomatic, the patient will require a transrectal ultrasound scan and multiple biopsies of the prostate.

He should not have been offered a PSA test if he was asymptomatic as there is no evidence to show that a national screening programme will bring more benefit than harm. With a positive biopsy result he would be offered a radical prostatectomy. In patients of advanced age or those who have significant life-limiting comorbidities and a life expectancy of less than 10 years, an 'active surveillance/watch and wait' protocol can be applied. Watchful waiting is a programme of regular examinations, PSA monitoring, and digital rectal examinations.

Androgen ablation has been used in situations in which patients are unwilling to undergo potentially curative treatment options yet want some form of treatment beyond watchful waiting. Androgen ablation can be performed medically or surgically. Examples of medical therapy include luteinizing hormone releasing hormone analogues (e.g. goserelin) or anti-androgens (e.g. bicalutamide). Surgical androgen ablation involves bilateral orchidectomy.

External-beam radiation therapy is used with curative intent for patients with clinically localized cancer and is often combined with androgen ablation.

Complications of external radiotherapy include cystitis, proctitis, enteritis, impotence, urinary retention and incontinence (7–10 per cent). Patients also exhibit the symptoms of androgen deprivation (e.g. decreased libido, impotence, hot flushes) if undergoing this form of therapy in conjunction with radiation therapy.

Finally, brachytherapy is a form of delivering radiation. It includes low-dose rate or high-dose rate brachytherapy. High-intensity frequency ultrasound is still in an experimental phase of development.

A 34-year-old man attends your clinic reporting that his twin brother has been diagnosed with prostate cancer.

J   Family screening is essential here as first-degree relatives of a man with prostate cancer diagnosed under the age of 50 are at far greater risk of developing prostate cancer themselves. All male siblings must be checked.

A 73-year-old man with prostate cancer attends your clinic complaining of new-onset back pain.

F   Regular follow-up of cancer patients is important to identify disease progression. PSA is a good tumour marker for monitoring this and a rise in PSA levels requires urgent investigation (CT scan of abdomen and pelvis, chest x-ray film, bone scan, positron emission tomography scan (PET), MRI spectroscopy). A PSA greater than 100 ng/mL is highly likely to be associated with bony metastases.

This patient has presented with possible bony metastases (secondaries). Plain x-ray may or may not reveal the classic osteosclerotic lesions; however, a radioisotope bone scan will show up hot spots where the metastatic deposits are located as radioisotope uptake occurs at these points.

A PET scan is an imaging study that uses cancer metabolism to illuminate cancer spread to other organs.

MRI spectroscopy combines anatomic information with metabolic activity to detect residual cancer in the gland.

This patient's disease progression would be discussed in a multidisciplinary team meeting and he may well be offered radiotherapy, but in the first instance he requires a bone scan and dexamethasone can be administered. Dexamethasone is a long-acting corticosteroid and is useful for reducing inflammatory oedema.

A 52-year-old man is diagnosed with prostate cancer and staging confirms the absence of secondary spread of disease.

A   This man is the ideal candidate for a laparoscopic radical prostatectomy (removal of the prostate and seminal vesicles). The goal is disease-free survival if the cancer is localized and is symptom-free survival if the cancer has spread outside the confines of the prostatic capsule. Typically, these patients are younger than 75 years, have very few comorbidities, with life expectancy longer than 10 years, and PSA levels less than 20 ng/mL. Patients must be consented for the risk of impotence, urinary incontinence and strictures.

55 Urinary incontinence (diagnosis/management)

ANSWERS: 1J, 2I, 3B, 4D, 5E

A 35-year-old woman presents 2 years after the birth of her child with urinary leakage on coughing, standing and sneezing.

J   Impaired urethral support from pelvic floor muscle weakness causes stress incontinence. Urine leakage is associated with increased abdominal pressure from laughing, sneezing, coughing, climbing stairs or other physical exertion.

First-line treatment for stress incontinence is pelvic floor exercises as recommended by NICE guidelines. Drug therapies are more useful in cases of urge incontinence. This is involuntary urine loss accompanied by a sudden strong desire to pass urine that is difficult to suppress, a result of uninhibited bladder contraction from detrusor hyperactivity caused by abnormalities of the CNS inhibitory pathway such as strokes and cervical stenosis, or from infection, stones or neoplasms.

Medications in the form of anticholinergic agents inhibit the binding of acetylcholine to the cholinergic receptor. This suppresses involuntary bladder contraction, increases the volume of the first involuntary bladder contraction, decreases the amplitude of the involuntary bladder contraction, and may increase bladder capacity.

Oxybutynin inhibits the action of acetylcholine on smooth muscle and has a direct antispasmodic effect on smooth muscle, thus increasing bladder capacity and decreasing uninhibited contractions.

A 25-year-old man presents with slowing of his urinary flow and terminal urethral dribbling. He has a past history of a treated sexually transmitted disease.

I   This patient is young so his bladder outlet symptoms, given his medical history, are likely to be due to a urethral stricture. The investigation of choice here is an urethrogram to diagnose and display the anatomy of the stricture.

A 75-year-old woman presents with recent onset of severe urinary urgency and bladder pain. Dipstix shows no nitrates, protein 1+ and blood 2+.

B   This patient is at risk of bladder cancer as the haematuria cannot be due to a urinary tract infection. Haematuria clinics are set up to assess the urinary tract by performing urine cytology, renal ultrasound, IVU or CT, and flexible cystoscopy. If all results are negative the patient can be reassured.

An 80-year-old man presents to the urology clinic with poor flow, frequency and nocturia. He is noted to have an elevated creatinine.

D   This man is describing symptoms of bladder outflow obstruction most likely due to an enlarged prostate. The degree of incomplete emptying can be assessed by ultrasound. The resultant back pressure on his kidneys is probably responsible for the elevated creatinine. Ultrasound of the kidneys is required to assess the degree of obstruction.

A 40-year-old woman who has had two previous colposuspensions for urinary incontinence now complains of mixed urge and stress leakage.

E   Mixed incontinence is characterized by detrusor overactivity and impaired urethral function (coexistence of stress and urge incontinence), involuntary loss of urine associated with urgency as well as exertion, cough, sneeze, or any effort that increase intra-abdominal pressure.

This patient has suffered from chronic urinary incontinence and her complex problem has been treated by surgery in the past but she remains symptomatic. Deciphering the aetiology of the symptoms is more important than offering treatment at this stage. Video urodynamics has the advantage of displaying the contraction and relaxation of the different sections of the urinary tract during the process of urination by fluoroscopy. It is useful for diagnosing detrusor–sphincter dyssynergia. This is a lack of coordination between the detrusor muscle and urethral sphincter such that the sphincter fails to relax when the detrusor contracts during bladder empty-ing. Post-void residual urine volume is assessed by catheterizing and measuring residual urine within 5 minutes after voiding. It determines the functional status of the lower urinary tract by reproducing the patient's symptoms.

Synchronous multichannel urodynamics measures and gives urody-namic parameters with radiographic visualization simultaneously. It is the most precise diagnostic study to evaluate micturition abnormalities of the lower urinary tract.

56 Management of renal stones

ANSWERS: 1G, 2I, 3H, 4A, 5F

A 40-year-old man has had a PCNL to treat a renal 2.5 cm stone. At the end of the procedure there is gross bleeding from the nephrostomy track. Nephrostomy tamponade fails to stop the bleeding.

G Renal stone disease affects men more than women in a ratio 3:1, with a lifetime risk of 2–3 per cent. The typical age is 30–50 years old with a 50 per cent risk of developing recurrent stones within the subsequent 10 years. The history is classic: 99 per cent of stones will be associated with at least microscopic haematuria, and family history is relevant. This patient is likely to have had an expedited or elective percutaneous nephrolithotomy. Patients are consented for stone recurrence, bleeding and failure to pass stone fragments. In this case the bleeding did not respond to nephrostomy tamponade (passage of nephrostomy tube to apply local pressure to stop bleeding); hence the next option, selective renal embolization, is attempted. This is a radiologically guided procedure to identify the bleeding vessel. If this fails, one would resort to open surgery to stop the bleeding.

A 35-year-old woman, in the first trimester of pregnancy, presents with severe right loin pain.

I Imaging is crucial, but an x-ray cannot be taken during the first tri-mester and so ultrasound scanning will be necessary to identify an obstructing calculus. This procedure is operator dependent and the results need interpreting by an experienced ultrasonographer. Note that the right ureter is often physiologically dilated in pregnancy.

A 50-year-old woman with diabetes presents with severe left loin pain, pyrexia, tachycardia and a white cell count of 24 000. Intravenous urogram shows no function on the initial 10-minute film.

H The working diagnosis is pyonephrosis which requires emergency decompression. This patient is diabetic and septic and her left kidney is completely obstructed. Percutaneous needle nephrostomy will divert the obstructed system until the stone either passes spontaneously or is managed electively by ESWL or PCNL.

A 37-year-old man presents with left renal colic. CT urogram shows a 5 mm stone in the lower third of the left ureter with moderate hydronephrosis.

A   Stones greater than 2 cm in size are usually confined to the kidney and will not pass the pelviureteric junction (PUJ), consequently requiring further intervention such as ESWL (in an unobstructed kidney) or PCNL. Stones smaller than 2 cm can pass the PUJ; but, they may get stuck causing PUJ obstruction requiring ureteric stent insertion to allow drainage of the kidney in order to preserve functioning renal tissue. Smaller stones will pass to the mid-ureter region, and stones smaller than 1 cm can pass to the lower third of the ureter. Stones of 5 mm or less in size will typically pass spontaneously, so this patient can be managed with simple analgesia and discharged home but needs outpatient follow-up to ensure stone passage by further imaging.

A 27-year-old man presents with severe loin pain. Plain x-ray shows a staghorn calculus.

F   A staghorn calculus is so-called for its shape which takes the form of the renal pelvis and pyramids resembling the horn of a stag. It is composed of a triple phosphate stone called struvite (calcium magnesium ammonium phosphate) which precipitates in alkaline urine. *Proteus* is a urea splitting organism (urease enzyme) and staghorn calculi are typically associated with *Proteus* infection.

The most important decision about management rests on the differential renal function. Chronic staghorn calculi result in poor renal function. If the function is less than 15 per cent then nephrectomy may be better than complicated stone treatment.

57 Lumps in the groin

Answers: 1D, 2B, 3A, 4E, 5K

An incidental lump is found during inguinal hernia repair. It is benign and left alone.

D   Lipoma of the cord is quite commonly found during hernia repair. It is a painless benign mass of fat cells that can recur if removed. With large lipomas some patients may feel that the surgery was not complete and would prefer to have had it removed.

A 60-year-old smoker complains of a throbbing lump in his right groin. Examination reveals an expansile pulsation in the mass.

B   An aneurysm is an abnormal dilatation of a blood vessel which presents clinically as an expansile, pulsatile mass. Common femoral artery aneurysms are usually caused by atherosclerotic disease. However, a false aneurysm can be caused by trauma to the vessel wall. If a patient is stabbed in the femoral artery, a haematoma develops outside the artery and eventually a thrombus occludes the hole in the arterial wall. The pressure in the artery may force this plug outwards into the haematoma to form a small cavity inside it.

A new significant groin lump is found in a 9-year-old boy who had previously undergone unsuccessful laparoscopy for undescended testis.

A   Undescended testes are investigated early and, if identified and viable, are brought down to the scrotum either by laparoscopy or open surgery. This is known as cryptorchidism and is a risk factor for testicular cancer. The main reason for surgery is in order to allow regular examination of the affected testicle. In this case the child's previous laparoscopy was unsuccessful, most likely due to the fact that the testicle was maldescended (located in a position along its normal developmental track but not in the scrotum). Note that if it is located outside the normal developmental track, this is called an 'ectopic testis'. By this age a maldescended testis will not contribute to fertility, which is normally adequate in the presence of a normal contralateral testis.

An 80-year-old man has been attending his GP for 3 years with an enlarging right-sided scrotal mass which disappears on lying flat but worsens during the day. The GP cannot get above the mass, nor does it transilluminate.

E   The mass described is most likely to be an inguinal hernia, although it could also be a varicocoele. A varicocoele is said to feel like 'a bag of worms', a hernia has a cough impulse. Examination of a hernia can sometimes reveal whether it is an indirect or direct inguinal hernia. *Direct* hernias push directly through the posterior wall of the inguinal canal and thus pressure over the internal ring after reduction will not stop it popping back through the wall. They often reduce easily and rarely strangulate.

Indirect inguinal hernias pass through the internal inguinal ring and therefore can be controlled by pressure over the internal inguinal ring after the hernia has been reduced. Generally speaking, direct inguinal hernias are not felt in the scrotum.

Femoral hernias are palpable below and lateral to the pubic tubercle, whereas inguinal hernias can be felt above and medial to this landmark. Femoral hernias are often irreducible and likely to strangulate.

A 69-year-old woman with right leg pain is diagnosed with a deep vein thrombosis on Doppler investigation. On examination there are firm rubbery matted masses in both groins.

K   Although direct pressure of a femoral aneurysm on the femoral vein can lead to venous obstruction and thrombosis, in this case the most likely answer is inguinal lymphadenopathy by the same pressure effect. The cause of the inguinal lymphadenopathy should be investigated.

58 Urological imaging/intervention

ANSWERS: 1J, 2K, 3I, 4E, 5D

A 45-year-old man has muscle-invasive transitional cell carcinoma of the bladder extending to multiple sites along the right ureter and involving the renal pelvis.

J   Filling defects can be seen on IVU, but in this case the diagnosis of muscle-invasive bladder disease is given indicating that retrograde urography has been performed. Cystoscopy is essential as 50 per cent of patients with upper urinary tract tumours have associated tumours in the bladder. Retrograde urography involves cannulation of the ureteric orifice at the time of cystoscopy and injection of contrast medium followed by x-ray imaging to look for a filling defect in the affected segment of ureter. Further management involves staging CT to look for the presence of distant metastases. Muscle-invasive disease involving the kidney, ureter and bladder requires radical treatment.

Thus the answer is that nephrocystourethrectomy and ileal conduit formation is the next step since the option of CT staging scan has not been given. Note the ratio of bladder to renal pelvis to ureteric urothelial tumour is 50:3:1, and ureteric disease has a tendency to multifocality.

An 83-year-old man with a PSA of 10 ng/mL and positive TRUS guided biopsy results denies lower urinary tract symptoms. He does not want any surgical intervention.

K   Management of his prostate cancer involves watchful waiting which is also known as active surveillance. This is disease monitoring with clinical examination and PSA testing and treatment of symptoms as and when they arise. HIFU is high-intensity focused ultrasound which is a minimally invasive form of treatment for prostate cancer but still requires a general anaesthetic and can cause some postoperative symptoms.

A 45-year-old man has raised PSA of 29 ng/mL and positive TRUS biopsy results. His brother died of prostate cancer aged 60 years.

I   This man has a positive family history. He needs full staging, followed by a radical prostatectomy, followed by radiotherapy as appropriate.

A 30-year-old man with a history of renal stones has been on a business trip and taken diclofenac and codeine throughout his meetings. He returns to attend A&E with further pain.

E   The investigation of choice here is ultrasound of the urinary tract. This
        man may well have an obstructed system and would need an urgent
        drainage, either in the form of a JJ stent or a nephrostomy to promote
        drainage. An ultrasound will show an obstructed system without the
        use of contrast and the degree of obstruction will indicate whether
        nephrostomy or JJ stent is more appropriate. It is important to appreci-
        ate urosepsis as he is young and tolerates the stress response better. His
        creatinine will be grossly deranged and, although he may be pain-free,
        he is likely to have loin tenderness.

        A 15-year-old female complains of severe loin pain when voiding.

D   The working diagnosis is vesico-ureteric reflux. The incompetent valve-
        like mechanism at the vesico-ureteric junction allows increases in blad-
        der pressure to be reflected to the kidneys, causing pain. This pain is
        apparent only during voiding and can be demonstrated on performing a
        micturating cystourethrogram. Treatment involves reimplantation of the
        ureters or subtrigonal injection of Polytef©, collagen or Macroplastique©
        into the ureteric orifices.

59 Renal masses/tumours

ANSWERS: 1C, 2K, 3H, 4F

        A 57-year-old man with acute cholecystitis undergoes ultrasound
        scanning of the abdomen. An incidental note of a renal lesion is
        made. The patient is informed and reassured that it is benign.

C   Simple cysts are the most common cystic renal lesion. They are usually
        asymptomatic and approximately one-third to one-half of people older
        than 50 years have one or more renal cysts. They are most commonly
        detected by ultrasound.

        If there is any evidence of calcifications, septa or multiple cysts which
        may obscure a carcinoma, renal CT scanning with contrast medium
        should be performed. Other cystic lesions can be Bosniak cysts, medul-
        lary sponge kidney (strongly associated with nephrolithiasis), acquired
        renal cystic disease seen in patients with end-stage renal failure, adult
        polycystic kidney disease, and renal cysts of Von Hippel-Lindau syn-
        drome (*VHL* is a tumour suppressor gene). Simple cysts are the only
        benign ones.

        A 46-year-old woman presents with a 3-month history of haema-
        turia, weight loss, fevers, lethargy and loin pain, and a palpable loin
        mass. She has no significant past medical history, or travel history.

K   Renal cell carcinoma presents as the classic triad of haematuria, loin pain
        and a palpable mass in only about 10 per cent of cases. Some present
        with 'clot colic' mimicking ureteric colic, but they can also present with

paraneoplastic syndromes or non-specifically as pyrexia of unknown origin. Hypercalcaemia occurs due to ectopic PTH-like hormone production and polycythaemia due to excess erythropoietin production.

A 23-year-old man attends A&E having fallen off a motorbike at 30 miles per hour. He presents with an expanding left loin mass, bruising and haematuria.

H   A thorough history of the presenting complaint is important for the differential diagnosis of any mass. In this case the history of trauma leads to the diagnosis of a haematoma.

A 37-year-old HIV-positive male presents to the clinic with haematuria, swinging pyrexia and raised white cell count. On examination he has a tender left loin mass.

F   There is almost always an associated clinical history when the symptoms of an inflammatory lesion are present. Patients with HIV infection are prone to abscess formation due to their immunosuppressed status, so unusual pathogens should be considered such as cryptococcosis, an encapsulated yeast which can be treated using amphotericin B. Note that immunosuppressed patients will often have blunted symptoms and do not necessarily present with the classic swinging pyrexia and raised white cell count from an abscess.

SECTION 5: EAR, NOSE AND THROAT SURGERY

QUESTIONS

60 Vertigo

A   Ménière's disease
B   vertebrobasilar insufficiency
C   hypercalcaemia
D   acute labyrinthitis
E   benign paroxysmal positional
    vertigo (BPPV)

F   acoustic neuroma
G   temporal arteritis
H   cholesteatoma
I   osteoarthritis of neck

For each clinical scenario below give the most likely cause for the clinical findings. Each option may be used only once.

1   A 50-year-old woman wakes in the middle of the night complaining of a spinning sensation with nausea that lasts for about 30 seconds. The symptoms are most obvious turning over onto the right side.

2   A 45-year-old man has a 4-month history of attacks of vertigo which lasts for hours associated with tinnitus and reduced hearing in the left ear. There is associated nausea.

3   A 38-year-old woman presents with severe vertigo and vomiting which lasts for days. There is no loss of hearing or tinnitus.

4   A 75-year-old man reports a chronic history of left-sided tinnitus and gradual hearing loss. He has recently been complaining of headaches and a sensation of unsteadiness when walking.

5   A 30-year-old woman presents with a history of chronic ear infections. She complains of an offensive discharge from her right ear with associated hearing loss for months. She has had severe vertigo for the last 48 hours.

Answers: see page 157

61 Sore throat

A   glandular fever
B   quinsy
C   chronic tonsillitis
D   acute tonsillitis
E   gastro-oesophageal reflux

F   foreign body in throat
G   lymphoma
H   squamous cell carcinoma of
tonsil

For each clinical scenario below give the most likely cause for the clinical
findings. Each option may be used only once.

1   A 20-year-old man presents with a 3-day history of a worsening sore throat
and raised temperature. He is complaining of right otalgia, difficulty opening
his mouth and a change in his speech. On examination he has trismus
(difficulty opening mouth), tonsil inflammation and soft palate swelling on the
right side. The uvula is deviated to the left.

2   An 18-year-old woman presents with a 7-day history of general malaise and
increasing throat pain, causing her difficulty in eating and drinking. On examination the tonsils are enlarged and inflamed with a sloughy exudate on the
surface. There is marked cervical lymphadenopathy. Full blood count shows a
lymphocytosis. Paul Bunnell test is positive.

3   A 24-year-old woman presents with a 3-day history of an increasing sore
throat, with general malaise and temperature. Examination reveals inflamed
enlarged tonsils with white spots. There is bilateral lymphadenopathy. Full
blood count shows a marked neutrophil leucocytosis. Paul Bunnell test is
negative.

4   A 50-year-old man presents with a daily sore throat, worse in the morning,
with no general malaise, temperature, dysphonia or dysphagia. This has
persisted for 2 months despite multiple courses of antibiotics.

5   A 70-year-old man presents with a 5-week history of right-sided sore throat
and worsening pain on swallowing. He has associated otalgia. He smokes 20
cigarettes every day and is known to be a heavy drinker.

Answers: see page 159

62 Nasal blockage

A	foreign bodies	E	nasal polyps
B	perennial allergic rhinitis	F	deviated nasal bones
C	rhinitis medicamentosa	G	Wegener's granulomatosis
D	deviated nasal septum	H	nasopharyngeal carcinoma

For each clinical scenario below give the most likely cause for the clinical findings. Each option may be used only once.

1   A 40-year-old known asthmatic presents with gradual blockage of both nostrils. The GP examined the nose and noted pale swellings in both nasal cavities. The patient is known to be sensitive to aspirin.

2   A 2-year-old child presents with a 1-week history of an offensive unilateral nasal discharge.

3   A 30-year-old woman presents with episodes of recurrent sneezing, watery rhinorrhoea and nasal blockage throughout the year. Her symptoms are worse at night.

4   A 40-year-old man presents with a history of bilateral nasal blockage. He has temporary relief with an 'over-the-counter' decongestant that he has been using for the last 2 months.

5   An 18-year-old man, who suffered nasal trauma, complains of a persistent right-sided nasal obstruction for 4 months following the assault.

Answers: see page 161

63 Hoarse voice

A   vocal cord granuloma
B   vocal cord nodules
C   hypercalcaemia
D   squamous cell carcinoma of
    larynx

E   vocal cord palsy
F   hypothyroidism
G   chronic laryngitis
H   carcinoma oesophagus

For each clinical scenario below give the most likely cause for the clinical findings. Each option may be used only once.

1   A 30-year-old lead singer of a rock band presents with a 2-month history of a hoarse voice. This is painless and there is no dysphagia.

2   A 45-year-old woman presents with a hoarse voice. She has taken numerous overdoses requiring admission to ITU and intubation.

3   A 75-year-old man presents with a 2-month history of a hoarse voice. He is a smoker of 20 cigarettes per day.

4   A 51-year-old woman complains of a hoarse voice following hemithyroidectomy.

5   A 48-year-old man presents with a 2-month history of hoarse voice. He takes oral antacid therapy for indigestion and denies any dysphagia.

Answers: see page 162

64 Dysphagia

A	foreign body	F	globus pharyngeus
B	pharyngeal pouch	G	thyroid goitre
C	oesphageal varices	H	motor neuron disease
D	hypopharyngeal carcinoma	I	oesophageal atresia
E	Mallory–Weiss syndrome	J	diffuse oesophageal spasm

For each clinical scenario below give the most likely cause for the clinical findings. Each option may be used only once.

1   A 70-year-old man presents with dysphagia and regurgitation of undigested food after about 5 minutes.

2   A 75-year-old woman presents with a 3-month history of increasing dysphagia to solids, pain on swallowing and weight loss.

3   A 35-year-old woman presents with a 3-month history of a sensation of a lump in the throat. There is no dysphagia and the sensation improves when she swallows.

4   A 50-year-old woman presents with a gradually increasing swelling in the lower part of the neck. Occasionally food can 'stick' when swallowed. The swelling was found to move on swallowing.

5   A 75-year-old man wakes up in the middle of the night with sudden onset of pain in the neck and difficulty swallowing his saliva. He has no symptoms during the day.

Answers: see page 164

65 Ear pain

A   acute suppurative otitis media
B   Ménière's disease
C   herpes zoster oticus
D   acute otitis externa
E   Kartagener's disease

F   temporomandibular joint
    dysfunction
G   malignant otitis externa
H   trigeminal neuralgia

For each clinical scenario below give the most likely cause for the clinical findings. Each option may be used only once.

1   A 30-year-old man presents with a 2-day history of severe right-sided earache after a recent holiday abroad. On examination there is marked tragal tenderness. The ear canal is swollen and filled with debris.

2   A 5-year-old boy with an upper respiratory tract infection had a 24-hour history of severe pain in his right ear followed by a pus-like discharge with resolution of pain.

3   A 72-year-old woman presents with severe left-sided ear pain followed by weakness to her face including eye closure. Vesicles are evident on her pinna.

4   A 40-year-old man has a 2-month history of intermittent right earache. There are no other ear symptoms. The pain is localized to the pre-auricular region. He is known to grind his teeth (bruxism) at night.

5   A 71-year-old diabetic patient presents with a 4-week history of severe left-sided earache. The pain radiates down his jaw and keeps him awake at night.

Answers: see page 165

66 Acute paediatric airway obstruction

A   laryngeal papillomatosis
B   foreign body
C   chronic obstructive airways
     disease
D   acute laryngotracheobronchitis
     (croup)

E   laryngomalacia
F   Down syndrome
G   acute epiglottitis
H   childhood asthma
I   acute tonsillitis

For each clinical scenario below give the most likely cause for the clinical findings. Each option may be used only once.

1   A 3-year-old boy presents with sudden-onset noisy breathing and drooling. He had a preceding upper respiratory tract infection and pyrexia. On examination the child appears frightened, flushed in the face, with inspiratory and expiratory stridor. There is indrawing of neck muscles and intercostals.

2   A 5-year-old girl with a 2-month history of a hoarse voice presents with worsening stridor over the last 72 hours. There is no associated temperature. This has been her third admission in just over a year with a similar problem.

3   A 2-year-old, whose brother is congenitally deaf, presents with a brief history of choking and cyanosis for about 10 seconds a few hours earlier. He is now completely asymptomatic.

4   A 4-year-old girl presents with a 24-hour history of general malaise and has developed a barking, noisy cough with difficulty in breathing. There is no drooling.

5   A 4-month-old baby presents with gradually worsening noisy breathing which is especially noticeable when she eats. She is on a lower centile for weight gain and has poor food intake.

Answers: see page 167

67 Swelling in the neck

A   branchial cyst
B   thyroid nodule
C   cervical rib
D   lymphoma
E   chemodectoma

F   sternomastoid tumour
G   dermoid cyst
H   pharyngeal pouch
I   thyroglossal cyst
J   cystic hygroma

For each clinical scenario below give the most likely cause for the clinical findings. Each option may be used only once.

1   A 43-year-old man presents to his GP with a 6-month history of a painless pulsatile mass at the angle of the jaw.

2   A 23-year-old girl complains of intermittent numbness and paraesthesia in her right hand for the past 2 months. On examination there is a fixed, hard, 1 cm × 2 cm swelling in the right supraclavicular fossa.

3   A 3-year-old boy is seen by his GP with an enlarging midline swelling that has been present for the past year. It is smooth and rounded, located just below the hyoid bone, measuring 2 cm × 2 cm, and rises on protrusion of the tongue.

4   A 32-year-old woman presents to her GP with a neck lump enlarging for the last 3 years. It measures 1 cm × 1.5 cm and is located behind the junction of the upper and middle thirds of the left sternocleidomastoid muscle. In the past this lump has become infected, resolving with oral antibiotics.

5   A 23-year-old man presents to his GP with a 2 cm × 3 cm painless lump at the angle of the jaw; it has been there for 2 months. He also complains of weight loss, night sweats and fever over the same period. Hepatosplenomegaly is detected on examination of the abdomen.

Answers: see page 168

68 Management of epistaxis

A   sphenopalatine artery ligation   F   topical nasal corticosteroid
B   nasal tampon   G   examination and cautery of nasal
C   anterior ethmoid artery ligation   septum
D   examination of post nasal space   H   maxillary artery ligation
E   saline douches

For each clinical scenario below give the most appropriate treatment for the clinical findings. Each option may be used only once.

1   A 75-year-old man presents with a profuse right-sided epistaxis lasting for 30 minutes which has not resolved with simple alar pressure.

2   A 15-year-old boy presents with a history of recurrent heavy left-sided epistaxis.

3   A 52-year-old man presents with several episodes of epistaxis a week lasting for several minutes. Examination of the nose reveals prominent vessels over Little's area.

4   A 25-year-old man is suffering from a profuse epistaxis after being punched in the nose. It has been bleeding for over 2 hours and has not resolved with alar pressure or packing.

Answers: see page 170

69 Nerves in ENT surgery

A	vagus nerve	I	glossopharyngeal nerve
B	vestibulocochlear nerve	J	accessory nerve
C	sympathetic plexus	K	chorda tympani
D	facial nerve	L	optic nerve
E	abducens nerve	M	hypoglossal nerve
F	trochlear nerve	N	brachial nerve injury
G	oculomotor nerve	O	phrenic nerve injury
H	olfactory nerve		

For each clinical scenario below suggest the most likely nerve involved. Each option may be used only once.

1   A 42-year-old man complains of a metallic taste in the mouth following myringoplasty (repair of ear drum).

2   A 35-year-old man is being treated on the ward for a severe right orbital cellulitis. On examination he has increasingly painful eye movements and in particular is unable to look to the right.

3   A 65-year-old man complains of stiffness in the shoulder after a lymph node biopsy from the neck.

4   A 75-year-old woman develops a chest infection several days following a tonsillectomy and neck dissection to treat a squamous cell carcinoma of the tonsil. Chest X ray shows significant elevation of the left hemidiaphragm.

Answers: see page 171

70 Parotid gland pathology

A   Mumps
B   Pleomorphic adenoma
C   Squamous cell carcinoma
D   Sialedenitis
E   Parotid gland abscess

F   Warthin's tumour
G   Sjögren's syndrome
H   Parotid haematoma
I   Frey's syndrome

1   An 85-year-old woman is brought to A&E from a nursing home with diffuse painful enlargement of the right parotid gland. Observations reveal a low-grade pyrexia.

2   A 28-year-old man presents with a discrete, smooth, firm 1.5 cm swelling over the tail of the right parotid gland. He feels that it has grown very slightly over the past 2 years. Fine needle aspiration reveals a mixture of epithelial, myoepithelial and stromal components.

3   A 38-year-old woman with a history of rheumatoid arthritis complains of persistently dry mouth and eyes.

4   A 95-year-old man presents with a necrotic swelling over the right cheek which is fungating through the skin.

Answers: see page 172

71 Complications of ENT surgery

A   Glossopharyngeal nerve injury   F   Septal perforation
B   Lingual nerve injury   G   CSF leak
C   Septal abscess   H   Hypoglossal nerve palsy
D   Trigeminal neuropraxia   I   Frey's syndrome
E   Chorda tympani avulsion

1   A 45-year-old woman complains of tongue numbness following excision of the right submandibular gland.

2   A 34-year-old woman complains of sweating over her cheek when she eats following surgery to remove a neck lump

3   A 46-year-old patient reports profuse constant watery discharge from the left nostril following endoscopic sinus surgery.

4   A 36-year-old patient complains of crusting and recurrent minor nose bleeds about a year after septal surgery.

Answers: see page 173

72 Congenital causes of deafness

A	Waardenburg syndrome	F	Refsum syndrome
B	Pierre Robin syndrome	G	Treacher Collins syndrome
C	Apert syndrome	H	Alport syndrome
D	Usher syndrome	I	Crouzon syndrome
E	Jervell and Lange-Nielson syndrome	J	Goldenhar syndrome
		K	Pendred syndrome

1   An 8-year-old girl with profound sensorineural deafness and a goitre.

2   A 3-year-old boy with hearing loss, craniostenosis, exophthalmos and a parrot beak nose.

3   A 10-year-old with haematuria and bilateral sensorineural hearing loss. There is a history of nephritis in the family.

4   A 5-year-old boy with sensorineural hearing loss and syncopal episodes during stress.

Answers: see page 174

ANSWERS

60 Vertigo

ANSWERS: 1E, 2A, 3D, 4F, 5H

A 50-year-old woman wakes in the middle of the night complaining of a spinning sensation with nausea that lasts for about 30 seconds. The symptoms are most obvious turning over onto the right side.

E   This woman has BPPV. The pathophysiology is under much debate, but detachment of calcium carbonate crystals (otoliths) that become detached from the utricle and saccule is perceived to be the likely pathology. The otoliths migrate to the posterior semicircular canal and stimulate the vestibular nerve on specific head movements. This causes a rotatory nystagmus. The diagnosis is confirmed with a positive Hallpike–Dix manoeuvre.

The patient is asked to sit upright with head facing the examiner. The examiner grasps the patient's head between his hands and rapidly moves the patient from a sitting to lying position with the head tipped below the horizontal plane, 45° to the side, and with the side of the affected ear (and semicircular canal) downwards. A positive test provokes vertigo and rotatory nystagmus that typically has a latency of a few seconds before onset and fatigues after about 30 seconds. If the nystagmus appears immediately on performing the manoeuvre and does not fatigue, a cerebellar mass lesion may be responsible and CT should be performed.

Treatment of BPPV is by an Epley repositioning procedure. A Hallpike manoeuvre is performed initially followed by stepwise rotations of the head to the opposite side before sitting the patient up. It is thought that this manoeuvre provides relief by dislodging otoliths from the posterior semicircular canal.

A 45-year-old man has a 4-month history of attacks of vertigo which lasts for hours associated with tinnitus and reduced hearing in the left ear. There is associated nausea.

A   Ménière's disease is characterized by a triad of recurrent symptoms including rotatory vertigo, tinnitus and loss of hearing in one ear alone. The vertigo can last for several hours. There may be preceding aural fullness or pressure sensation. There is often associated nausea or vomiting. The cause of the condition is unknown. Repeat audiograms may show a unilateral fluctuating hearing loss. Treatment is dependent on the severity and frequency of attacks. Vestibular sedatives (e.g. prochlorperazine) are taken for acute episodes. Prophylactic treatment includes advice with regard to low salt and caffeine intake and pharmacological intervention with betahistine (labyrinthine vasodilator). The condition is normally self-limiting. There is a 50 per cent chance it may develop in the other ear. Surgery is indicated only in carefully selected severe cases and includes grommet insertion with administration of drugs (e.g. gentamicin) to ablate vestibular function, and endolymphatic surgery (though there are mixed results on the benefit of this).

A 38-year-old woman presents with severe vertigo and vomiting which lasts for days. There is no loss of hearing or tinnitus.

D   Acute labyrinthitis usually has a viral infective origin and is often preceded by an upper respiratory tract infection. There is a sudden onset of rotatory vertigo, nausea and vomiting. Symptom severity can result in the patient being confined to bed for days. Treatment involves the use of vestibular sedatives (e.g. prochlorperazine). Hospital admission is sometimes necessary for cases of intractable vomiting.

A 75-year-old man reports a chronic history of left-sided tinnitus and gradual hearing loss. He has recently been complaining of head-aches and a sensation of unsteadiness when walking.

F   Acoustic neuroma is a rare, benign, slow-growing tumour of the VIII cranial nerve which rarely presents with vertigo. It more often presents with unilateral tinnitus and deafness (rarely sudden-onset). Large tumours may cause facial pain, numbness and paraesthesia through trigeminal nerve stimulation. Any asymmetrical cochlear symptoms require investigation for this condition with an MRI scan. If the acoustic neuroma is small a watch and wait policy can be adopted with serial MRI scans. Treatment options include surgery or radiotherapy.

A 30-year-old woman presents with a history of chronic ear infec-tions. She complains of an offensive discharge from her right ear with associated hearing loss for months. She has had severe vertigo for the last 48 hours.

H   Cholesteatoma is a complication of chronic ear infection due to squamous epithelium invading the middle ear ('skin in the middle ear') and is not a tumour as the name suggests. It occurs in the region of the pars flaccida of the ear drum and erodes the bone above this area called the 'attic region'. There is typically a chronic offensive discharge from the ear and hearing loss.

The cholesteatoma can erode the temporal bone and structures within it including the ossicles, facial nerve and the lateral semicircular canal. An erosion of the lateral semicircular canal is called a fistula and can result in sudden-onset vertigo. This requires urgent surgical treatment to remove the cholesteatoma and place a patch (e.g. temporalis fascia) over the hole.

Other complications of cholesteatoma include intracranial infections (e.g. meningitis), extradural, subdural and intracerebral abscesses, and lateral sinus thrombosis.

61 Sore throat

ANSWERS: 1B, 2A, 3D, 4E, 5H

A 20-year-old man presents with a 3-day history of a worsening sore throat and raised temperature. He is complaining of right otalgia, difficulty opening his mouth and a change in his speech. On examination he has trismus (difficulty opening mouth), tonsil inflammation and soft palate swelling on the right side. The uvula is deviated to the left.

B   This man has a right-sided quinsy. This is due to a collection of pus around the fibrous capsule of the tonsil causing the soft palate to bulge. Aspiration of this pus under topical anaesthesia is usually performed as it can dramatically improve the significant symptoms. Antibiotic therapy is commenced depending on local protocols (usually a cephalosporin plus anaerobic cover with metronidazole). Trismus occurs due to inflammation involving the pterygoid muscles which open and close the mouth. Patients with recurrent quinsy should be considered for tonsillectomy.

An 18-year-old woman presents with a 7-day history of general malaise and increasing throat pain, causing her difficulty in eating and drinking. On examination the tonsils are enlarged and inflamed with a sloughy exudate on the surface. There is marked cervical lymphadenopathy. Full blood count shows a lymphocytosis. Paul Bunnell test is positive.

A   This is a presentation of infectious mononucleosis which is commonly known as glandular fever. It is an infection caused by the Epstein–Barr virus. It can also affect other organs (e.g. liver) causing hepatomegaly. It most commonly affects teenagers and presents with general malaise, sore throat, dysphagia and occasionally upper airway obstruction due to massive enlargement of the tonsils. There may be significant lymphadenopathy in the neck and possibly hepatosplenomegaly on abdominal examination. A Paul Bunnell (monospot) blood test can confirm the diagnosis (this may be negative initially). Treatment is typically with i.v. antibiotics and steroids if there is any sign of airway obstruction. There is a risk of developing a maculopapular rash if ampicillin is administered. Patients should be warned to avoid alcohol due to hepatic involvement and contact sports should also be avoided for at least 6 weeks after infection as the enlarged organs (liver/spleen) are at risk of injury.

A 24-year-old woman presents with a 3-day history of an increasing sore throat, with general malaise and temperature. Examination reveals inflamed, enlarged tonsils with white spots. There is bilateral lymphadenopathy. Full blood count shows a marked neutrophil leucocytosis. Paul Bunnell test is negative.

D   Acute tonsillitis presents with a sore throat, general malaise and reduced oral intake. Examination confirms enlarged, erythematous tonsils with pus within the tonsillar crypts. The upper cervical chain of nodes is typically enlarged (jugulodigastric). Causative organisms include viruses (e.g. influenza, parainfluenza and adenovirus) and bacteria (e.g. *Streptococcus* and *Haemophilus*). Treatment is with penicillin-based antibiotic therapy, antipyretics and fluids for rehydration. Surgery is recommended for recurrent attacks.

A 50-year-old man presents with a daily sore throat, worse in the morning, with no general malaise, temperature, dysphonia or dysphagia. This has persisted for 2 months despite multiple courses of antibiotics.

E   Gastro-oesophageal reflux presents with a burning sensation in the chest. It can also present with throat symptoms including hoarse voice, sensation of a lump in the throat (globus pharyngeus) and sore throat. Examination of the oropharynx and lower pharynx with a flexible nasendoscope is usually normal, though there may be some erythema around the posterior aspect of the larynx (arytenoids). Risk factors include alcohol, hiatus hernia, obesity and large meals late at night.

Treatment includes conservative measures to address these risk factors. Medical therapy involves use of proton pump inhibitors and regular antacids. Surgery is reserved for patients with severe symptoms which are resistant to medical treatment (e.g. laparoscopic fundoplication).

A 70-year-old man presents with a 5-week history of right-sided sore throat and worsening pain on swallowing. He has associated otalgia. He smokes 20 cigarettes every day and is known to be a heavy drinker.

H   Squamous cell carcinoma of the tonsil presents in adults with persistent unilateral throat pain and painful swallowing (odynophagia) often with referred otalgia to the same side. Risk factors include smoking and excessive alcohol consumption. Metastases can occur to nodes in the neck. The tonsil is enlarged and often ulcerated on the affected side. There may be palpable neck nodes.

Treatment is dependent on the stage of the tumour and may include surgery combined with radiotherapy. Large tumours may require some reconstruction of the pharyngeal defect with a free flap (e.g. radial forearm).

62 Nasal blockage

ANSWERS: 1E, 2A, 3B, 4C, 5D

A 40-year-old known asthmatic presents with gradual blockage of both nostrils. The GP examined the nose and noted pale swellings in both nasal cavities. The patient is known to be sensitive to aspirin.

E   Nasal polyps are non-neoplastic swellings arising from the lining of the sinus mucosa. Their aetiology is currently unknown, although studies have postulated allergic, genetic or infective (particularly fungal) causes. At present there is no definitive curative therapy.

Nasal polyps typically present with symptoms of chronic rhinosinusitis (nasal blockage, rhinorrhoea, post nasal drip) and loss of smell (anosmia). Sampter's triad refers to the presence of nasal polyps, asthma and aspirin allergy.

Treatment includes topical steroids (either nasal sprays or short courses of steroid nose drops) and antihistamines. Oral steroids can be very effective at reducing the size of nasal polyps but due to the side-effect profile can be taken only for limited periods. Surgery is reserved for patients who have failed medical treatment and include simple nasal polypectomy or functional endoscopic sinus surgery, whereby the polyps are removed and sinus drainage is improved.

A 2-year-old child presents with a 1-week history of an offensive unilateral nasal discharge.

A   Any child who presents with a unilateral nasal discharge must be considered to have a foreign body until proven otherwise. They may need to have an examination of their nose under a general anaesthetic.

A 30-year-old woman presents with episodes of recurrent sneezing, watery rhinorrhoea and nasal blockage throughout the year. Her symptoms are worse at night.

B   Perennial allergic rhinitis is an IgE-mediated type 1 hypersensitivity reaction to allergens all year round. The most common allergens are house dust mites (HDM) which are prevalent in the bedroom, particularly on pillows, bedding and carpeted floors. Patients complain of watery rhinorrhoea, sneezing and watery itchy eyes. In the case of HDM allergy, symptoms are worse at night in bed. Skin prick allergen testing or a blood test (RAST: radioallergosorbent test) can be used to aid diagnosis. Seasonal allergic rhinitis is better known as hay fever.

Treatment is multimodal and includes allergy avoidance measures, topical steroid nasal treatment, oral antihistamines, intramuscular steroids, and desensitization with serial injection of small amounts of allergens (in a controlled environment as there is potential risk of anaphylaxis). Surgery is rarely indicated. Shrinkage of the lining of the nose (diathermy to inferior turbinates) may temporarily help with nasal blockage.

A 40-year-old man presents with a history of bilateral nasal blockage. He has temporary relief with an 'over-the-counter' decongestant that he has been using for the last 2 months.

C   Rhinitis medicamentosa is where the lining of the nose (inferior turbinates) swells up and causes nasal obstruction through the prolonged use of nasal vasoconstrictors (e.g. xylometazoline drops). It is thought to occur due to a 'rebound' vasodilatation of the blood vessels within the lining of the nose. It is recommended that people should not take topical nasal decongestants for more than 1 week.

An 18-year-old man, who suffered nasal trauma, complains of a persistent right-sided nasal obstruction for 4 months following the assault.

D   The nasal septum forms the central support of the nose. It is composed of cartilage anteriorly and bone inferiorly and posteriorly. It may be fractured through trauma or deviation may develop congenitally. Patients complaining of nasal blockage particularly on the side of the bend may benefit from surgery (septoplasty) where part of the septum is removed to allow it to align more centrally. Deviated nasal bones alone do not often cause obstructive symptoms. Performing a rhinoplasty would improve the cosmesis in this situation.

63 Hoarse voice

ANSWERS: 1B, 2A, 3D, 4E, 5G

A 30-year-old lead singer of a rock band presents with a 2-month history of a hoarse voice. This is painless and there is no dysphagia.

B   Vocal cord nodules arise from vocal misuse and are otherwise known as 'singer's' or 'screamer's' nodules. They are painless, normally bilateral and affect the anterior part of the larynx. This is the most common cause of a hoarse voice in children. Treatment is conservative with speech and language therapy.

A 45-year-old woman presents with a hoarse voice. She has taken numerous overdoses requiring admission to ITU and intubation.

A   Vocal cord granulomas are non-neoplastic swellings affecting the posterior part of the laryngeal framework (arytenoid cartilages) and can be unilateral or bilateral. They occur as a result of chronic trauma particularly with contact through prolonged intubation on ITU. Treatment is conservative through voice therapy, though the patient may need to have a diagnostic microlaryngoscopy and biopsy under a general anaesthetic.

A 75-year-old man presents with a 2-month history of a hoarse voice. He is a smoker of 20 cigarettes per day.

D   Squamous cell carincoma of the larynx is the commonest head and neck cancer in the western world. Its incidence increases with age, presenting most commonly in the seventh decade, with males affected more than females. Smokers and alcohol drinkers are at increased risk of developing this disease.

Any unexplained persistent hoarseness lasting more than 6 weeks requires urgent referral to an ENT specialist. Squamous cell carcinomas of the vocal cords normally present early because small tumours cause hoarseness. As they increase in size they can cause difficulty in breathing (particularly symptoms of stridor) and dysphagia through involvement of the pharynx and spread to lymph nodes in the neck. Treatment is dependent on the size of the tumour and includes radiotherapy for small lesions and surgery (e.g. laryngectomy) for larger tumours.

A 51-year-old woman complains of a hoarse voice following hemi-thyroidectomy.

E   The recurrent laryngeal nerve is the main motor supply for the muscles of the larynx. The left nerve descends into the chest before returning into the neck to enter the larynx. In this way a patient with a left-sided vocal cord palsy may have chest pathology (e.g. lung malignancy) as a potential cause. Other causes include other malignancies (e.g. oesophagus, thyroid), iatrogenic from thyroid surgery, and penetrating trauma.

Unilateral palsy may present with hoarseness and a weak cough (bovine). This may be treated with speech and language therapy to strengthen the mobile side, or with surgery to allow the opposite side of the larynx to meet the paralysed side (Teflon injection of paralysed cord; medialization of the paralysed cord, e.g. thyroplasty). If there is a bilateral cord palsy the patient may present with stridor and an emergency tracheostomy may be warranted in order to stabilize the airway.

A 48-year-old man presents with a 2-month history of hoarse voice. He takes oral antacid therapy for indigestion and denies any dysphagia.

G   The aetiology of chronic laryngitis is thought to be multifactorial including smoking, vocal abuse and gastro-oesophageal reflux. In its milder form the vocal cords are inflamed. In more extreme forms there is marked oedema and swelling known as Reinke's oedema. Initial treatment involves addressing risk factors (e.g. smoking cessation combined with voice therapy). In more severe cases of Reinke's oedema, surgery can be performed to remove the oedematous matrix of the vocal cord.

64 Dysphagia

ANSWERS: 1B, 2D, 3F, 4G, 5A

A 70-year-old man presents with dysphagia and regurgitation of undigested food after about 5 minutes.

B A pharyngeal pouch is a diverticulum of the mucosa of the posterior pharyngeal wall between a weak area of musculature called Killian's dehiscence. It presents with increasing dysphagia and regurgitation of undigested food. As a result there may be a history of aspiration pneumonia as food spills into the airway. Barium swallow is the diagnostic investigation of choice. There is approximately a 1 per cent risk of squamous cell carcinoma present in the wall of the pouch.

In patients with minimal symptoms no specific treatment is necessary. In severe cases surgery is recommended, which includes endoscopic stapling of the dividing wall of the pouch and oesophagus, or excision via an external neck incision in cases where stapling cannot be done or has failed.

A 75-year-old woman presents with a 3-month history of increasing dysphagia to solids, pain on swallowing and weight loss.

D Hypopharyngeal carcinoma presents with progressive dysphagia from solids to liquids. Dysphonia occurs through direct invasion into the larynx or vocal cord palsy. Lymph node metastases are common. There may be anorexia and weight loss in advanced disease. Prognosis is generally poor (a 40 per cent 1-year survival rate).

Treatment is dependent on a number of factors including site and extent of disease. The options include radiotherapy, surgery, a combination of both, or palliation. Surgery involves tumour resection and reconstruction of the defect with grafts (pectoralis major, radial forearm free flap, gastric transposition). The neck is treated with either radiotherapy or neck dissection. As with all cases of head and neck cancer there is a multidisciplinary approach throughout the care, which needs to be continued after initial recovery and discharge from hospital.

A 35-year-old woman presents with a 3-month history of a sensation of a lump in the throat. There is no dysphagia and the sensation improves when she swallows.

F Globus pharyngeus is the sensation of a 'lump in the throat'. There is no dysphagia or pain on swallowing. The symptom is intermittent and can seem worse when the patient is anxious. Gastro-oesophageal reflux may play a role although this is not proven. ENT examination is normal. There is no specific treatment indicated except reassurance. The more anxious patient may need a barium swallow or examination of the upper oesophagus under general anaesthetic just to allay concerns.

A 50-year-old woman presents with a gradually increasing swelling in the lower part of the neck. Occasionally food can 'stick' when swallowed. The swelling was found to move on swallowing.

G   An enlarged thyroid gland (goitre) can cause dysphagia by pressure effects on the oesophagus which lies posterior to the trachea. This can occur particularly in cases of retrosternal extension. These are indications for surgery. A rapidly enlarging gland with dysphonia raises the possibility of an anaplastic cancer or lymphoma.

A 75-year-old man wakes up in the middle of the night with sudden onset of pain in the neck and difficulty swallowing his saliva. He has no symptoms during the day.

A   The most likely cause is a swallowed denture plate. With a large plate the patient may have difficulty swallowing saliva. Pain is a main feature.

A lateral soft tissue neck x-ray may show part of the plate if radio-opaque. Other findings such as increased prevertebral shadowing of air in the oesophagus may also be seen on the plain x-ray. A barium swallow would show a filling defect.

Management is urgent removal with a rigid endoscope under a general anaesthetic. Delay may risk a perforation of the oesophagus. Mediastinitis is a serious complication of oesophageal perforation which has a high mortality rate. Symptoms of perforation include chest pain which radiates through to the interscapular region. There may also be signs of shock including tachycardia and hypotension as well as pyrexia. Surgical emphysema is palpable in the neck. Intravenous antibiotics need to be administered and the advice of a thoracic surgeon should be sought.

65 Ear pain

ANSWERS: 1D, 2A, 3C, 4F, 5G

A 30-year-old man presents with a 2-day history of severe right-sided earache after a recent holiday abroad. On examination there is marked tragal tenderness. The ear canal is swollen and filled with debris.

D   Otitis externa is inflammation within the external auditory meatus. Risk factors include cotton bud usage, water exposure, eczema and diabetes.

The most common organism is *Pseudomonas aeruginosa*. Treatment includes topical antibiotic and steroid ear drops and aural toilet. In cases of marked oedema of the ear canal, insertion of a sponge wick allows the antibiotic drops to penetrate to the deeper part of the canal. Chronic ear drop use should be discouraged as it may lead to fungal infection (e.g. *Aspergillus niger*) with visible spores and hyphae.

A 5-year-old boy with an upper respiratory tract infection had a 24-hour history of severe pain in his right ear followed by a pus-like discharge with resolution of pain.

A   Acute otitis media is infection within the middle ear space. It is more common in children and may present with otalgia and general malaise following an upper respiratory tract infection. The tympanic membrane can rupture due to a build-up of pus in the middle ear – alleviating the pain but resulting in a purulent discharge. In very small children the symptoms may be more non-specific with poor feeding, irritability and pyrexia.

The most common organisms include *Streptococcus pneumoniae* and *Haemophilus influenzae*. Treatment includes antibiotics, analgesics and antipyretics. Complications can arise albeit rarely and include mastoiditis, meningitis and intracranial abscesses.

A 72-year-old woman presents with severe left-sided ear pain followed by weakness to her face including eye closure. Vesicles are evident on her pinna.

C   Herpes zoster oticus (Ramsay Hunt syndrome) is a viral infection which causes vesicles on the pinna or external auditory meatus, lower motor neuron VII nerve palsy and marked otalgia. This is more common in the elderly. Treatment includes steroids, aciclovir and eye care (regular drops, ointment and an eye patch at night if unable to close the eyelids fully to prevent corneal abrasion).

A 40-year-old man has a 2-month history of intermittent right earache. There are no other ear symptoms. The pain is localized to the pre-auricular region. He is known to grind his teeth (bruxism) at night.

F   Temporomandibular joint dysfunction can present with referred otalgia. There may be a history of trauma to the joint (strained during yawning or chewing) or teeth grinding (bruxism). There is often associated muscular spasm. Treatment options include drugs (NSAIDs, benzodiazepines), dental splints, steroid injections and joint surgery.

A 71-year-old diabetic patient presents with a 4-week history of severe left-sided earache. The pain radiates down his jaw and keeps him awake at night.

G   The term 'malignant otitis externa' is a misnomer as there is no malignancy. There is significant inflammation affecting the floor of the ear canal due to osteitis. It typically affects elderly diabetics and presents with intractable earache which can radiate to the jaw. Cranial nerve palsies (most commonly the facial nerve) in this clinical situation clinch the diagnosis. The most common organism is *Pseudomonas aeruginosa*. Treatment includes long-term antibiotics (e.g. ciprofloxacin), regular aural toilet and (if diabetic) close control of blood sugar level.

66 Acute paediatric airway obstruction

ANSWERS: 1G, 2A, 3B, 4D, 5E

A 3-year-old boy presents with sudden-onset noisy breathing and drooling. He had a preceding upper respiratory tract infection and pyrexia. On examination the child appears frightened, flushed in the face, with inspiratory and expiratory stridor. There is indrawing of neck muscles and intercostals.

G   Acute epiglottitis is a life-threatening medical emergency. The priority is to stabilize the child's airway while causing minimal distress. This requires effective multidisciplinary input including a senior anaesthetist, paediatrician and ENT surgeon. The child should be transferred to an anaesthetic room with a view to endotracheal intubation. Intravenous antibiotics and steroids are commenced. *Haemophilus influenzae* type B is the most common causative organism, though the introduction of vaccination has resulted in a significant reduction in incidence of acute epiglottitis.

A 5-year-old girl with a 2-month history of a hoarse voice presents with worsening stridor over the last 72 hours. There is no associated temperature. This has been her third admission in just over a year with a similar problem.

A   Laryngeal papillomatosis is characterized by benign wart-like lesions which can affect any part of the respiratory tract. The causative organisms are human papillomavirus types 6 and 11. Maternal transmission by mothers affected with genital warts through vaginal birth is believed to be the main source of infection.

Presenting symptoms include abnormal cry, dysphonia and stridor in advanced cases. Treatment requires laser excision of differing intervals. Tracheostomy is not recommended because of the risk of implantation of papilloma into trachea and bronchi. Medical treatments include alpha-interferon and retinoic acid.

A 2-year-old, whose brother is congenitally deaf, presents with a brief history of choking and cyanosis for about 10 seconds a few hours earlier. He is now completely asymptomatic.

B   The presentation of a foreign body in the airway is dependent on its size and whether the foreign body is organic or corrosive (e.g. a hearing aid battery). A small non-organic foreign body may present with a brief episode of choking, cyanosis and little else. There may be occlusion of a bronchus with subsequent collapse of a lobe causing shortness of breath. A large foreign body may result in occlusion of the airway at the level of the larynx with laryngospasm resulting in death. Organic foreign bodies (e.g. peanut) can cause marked inflammation in the lower airways due to the oil irritating the mucosa. Removal via a bronchoscope can be quite challenging as the peanut tends to fragment into small pieces.

A 4-year-old girl presents with a 24-hour history of general malaise and has developed a barking, noisy cough with difficulty in breathing. There is no drooling.

D   Acute laryngotracheobronchitis (croup) presents with inspiratory stridor and a barking cough. Inflammation involves the lower respiratory tract particularly in the subglottis. Treatment includes antibiotics and steam inhalation. In severe cases hospital admission is required for close observation, including administration of steroids and nebulized adrenaline. In rare cases the airway needs stabilizing with endotracheal intubation.

A 4-month-old baby presents with gradually worsening noisy breathing which is especially noticeable when she eats. She is on a lower centile for weight gain and has poor food intake.

E   Laryngomalacia can present soon after birth. It is the most common cause of stridor in infants. There is infolding of the epiglottis (floppy epiglottis) into the airway on inspiration. This is normally a self-limiting condition, but if the stridor becomes severe with signs of respiratory distress (indrawing of intercostals and use of accessory muscles) and affected feeding, surgery is recommended to improve the airway.

67 Swelling in the neck

ANSWERS: 1E, 2C, 3I, 4A, 5D

A 43-year-old man presents to his GP with a 6-month history of a painless pulsatile mass at the angle of the jaw.

E   A chemodectoma is a benign tumour arising from neural crest cells of the carotid body at the junction of the bifurcation of the carotid. A pulsatile mass is present which moves in a lateral but not vertical direction and has a bruit on auscultation. Angiography shows widening of the carotid bifurcation (known as the lyre sign). Ten per cent of tumours are malignant, 10 per cent familial and 10 per cent secrete catecholamines. Surgery is the main treatment, though radiotherapy is indicated in patients not suitable for surgery.

A 23-year-old girl complains of intermittent numbness and paraesthesia in her right hand for the past 2 months. On examination there is a fixed, hard, 1 cm × 2 cm swelling in the right supraclavicular fossa.

C A cervical rib is a supernumerary rib which arises from the costal part of the seventh cervical vertebra. It occurs above the first rib and may press on neurovascular structures including the brachial plexus and subclavian artery. It can present as a hard mass in the posterior triangle with concomitant upper limb symptoms including paraesthesia, pain and weakness.

A 3-year-old boy is seen by his GP with an enlarging midline swelling that has been present for the past year. It is smooth and rounded, located just below the hyoid bone, measuring 2 cm × 2 cm, and rises on protrusion of the tongue.

I A thyroglossal cyst is a swelling resulting from a failure of obliteration of the embryological tract of the thyroid gland. The thyroid arises from the foramen caecum at the base of the tongue and descends into the lower anterior neck intimately related to the hyoid bone. It can present as a painless swelling in the anterior triangle, typically in the midline, or, if infected, as an erythematous painful swelling. It moves on tongue protrusion and swallowing because of its relationship with the hyoid bone. It is the most common cause of an anterior neck swelling in children. Treatment is excision of cyst and tract including a portion of the hyoid bone (Sistrunk's operation).

A 32-year-old woman presents to her GP with a neck lump enlarging for the last 3 years. It measures 1 cm × 1.5 cm and is located behind the junction of the upper and middle thirds of the left sternocleidomastoid muscle. In the past this lump has become infected, resolving with oral antibiotics.

A A branchial cyst is a neck swelling which is thought to arise from either the embryological remnants of first and third pharyngeal pouches, or from cystic degeneration within a lymph node. The cyst presents in young adults at the anterior border of sternocleidomastoid at the junction of the upper one-third and lower two-thirds. The swelling may enlarge rapidly and become painful if infected. Surgical excision is recommended when the infection has settled.

A 23-year-old man presents to his GP with a 2 cm × 3 cm painless lump at the angle of the jaw; it has been there for 2 months. He also complains of weight loss, night sweats and fever over the same period. Hepatosplenomegaly is detected on examination of the abdomen.

D   A lymphoma is a malignant tumour made up of lymphoid cells. This can present with persistently or fluctuating enlargement of lymph nodes in patients between 20 and 30 years of age. There may be type A symptoms including weight loss, night sweats and poor appetite. Incisional biopsy is recommended. CT staging scans include neck, chest, abdomen and pelvis. Treatment is in the form of chemotherapy.

Two main subtypes exist: Hodgkin's (20–25 per cent of all lymphomas) and non-Hodgkin's (75–80 per cent). The former is diagnosed histologically with the presence of Reed–Sternberg cells. Either T-cells or B-cells are affected.

68 Management of epistaxis

ANSWERS: 1B, 2D, 3G, 4C

A 75-year-old man presents with a profuse right-sided epistaxis lasting for 30 minutes which has not resolved with simple alar pressure.

B   Epistaxis should be initially managed with simple first aid measures in the first instance. Firm continuous alar pressure (pinching the nose) for at least 15 minutes with the patient's head leaning forward will terminate most simple nose bleeds. In this case there is active bleeding despite alar pressure and therefore a nasal tampon is indicated to apply more effective tamponade against the bleeding area. Nasal tampons expand when brought into contact with fluid and close up the dead space within the nasal airway allowing pressure against the bleeding vessel.

A 15-year-old boy presents with a history of recurrent heavy left-sided epistaxis.

D   Most epistaxes have a simple cause, e.g. trauma, idiopathic, and do not require detailed investigation. Recurrent heavy unilateral epistaxis in an adolescent male is an indication for an endoscopic examination of the post nasal space to rule out a juvenile angiofibroma. This is a benign vascular tumour arising from near the sphenopalatine foramen typically in adolescent males. It is associated with symptoms of unilateral nasal obstruction and recurrent severe unilateral epistaxis.

A 52-year-old man presents with several episodes of epistaxis a week lasting for several minutes. Examination of the nose reveals prominent vessels over Little's area.

G   Little's area is the name given to a highly vascular area on the anterior inferior aspect of the nasal septum. It represents an anastomosis of several arterial branches from the internal and external carotid arteries. Contributing vessels include branches from the sphenopalatine artery, greater palatine artery, anterior ethmoidal artery and superior labial artery. It is the most common site of anterior epistaxis and therefore cauterising this area with silver nitrate/diathermy can be an effective treatment.

A 25-year-old man is suffering from a profuse epistaxis after being punched in the nose. It has been bleeding for over 2 hours and has not resolved with alar pressure or packing.

C   This is a scenario where there is persistent severe bleeding following trauma to the nose that has not resolved with packing the nose. If there is an obviously displaced nasal fracture, then reduction of the nasal fracture may sometimes stop the bleeding. If this does not help then it is likely that a branch of the anterior ethmoidal artery has been cut and the most advisable course of action would be to ligate the anterior ethmoidal artery under general anaesthetic as a matter of urgency.

69 Nerves in ENT surgery

ANSWERS: 1K, 2E, 3J, 4O

A 42-year-old man complains of a metallic taste in the mouth following myringoplasty (repair of ear drum).

K   The chorda tympani runs just beneath the tympanic membrane and can be traumatized/severed during middle ear surgery. It carries afferent fibres of taste from the anterior two-thirds of the tongue and efferent parasympathetic secretomotor fibres from the inferior salivary nucleus to the submandibular and sublingual glands. It is more common for the patient to report abnormal tastes in the mouth e.g. metallic taste rather than complete loss of taste following ipsilateral nerve injury.

A 35-year-old man is being treated on the ward for a severe right orbital cellulitis. On examination he has increasingly painful eye movements and in particular is unable to look to the right.

E   Severe orbital cellulitis secondary to paranasal sinusitis may be complicated by cavernous sinus thrombosis. This is usually due to retrograde spread of infection via the superior and inferior ophthalmic veins. Several cranial nerves course through the cavernous sinus including III, IV, V (ophthalmic and maxillary divisions) and VI. The abducens nerve is most commonly affected clinically. The abducens nerve supplies the lateral rectus muscle of the eye and therefore nerve injury results in impairment of lateralizing/abducting the eye.

A 65-year-old man complains of stiffness in the shoulder after a lymph node biopsy from the neck.

J   The accessory nerve is at risk of injury when removing a lymph node from the posterior triangle of the neck. Early indications of neuropraxia include stiffness of the shoulder rather than complete inability to shrug the shoulder. Early physiotherapy is indicated to reduce the risk of long-term stiffness and an iatrogenic frozen shoulder.

A 75-year-old woman develops a chest infection several days following a tonsillectomy and neck dissection to treat a squamous cell carcinoma of the tonsil. Chest x-ray shows significant elevation of the right hemidiaphragm.

O   The phrenic nerve provides the only motor supply to the diaphragm and therefore injury to the nerve will result in paralysis of the ipsilateral hemidiaphragm. In many patients this will be asymptomatic but in the postoperative period there is a risk of atelectasis and consequent lower respiratory tract infection. This is particularly pertinent for patients with head and neck cancer that may be heavy smokers with chronic obstructive pulmonary disease (COPD) putting them further at risk of infection. Nerve repair should be carried out at the time of surgery if it is recognized. If the nerve injury is only discovered postoperatively early chest physiotherapy is useful to reduce the risk of chest infection.

70 Parotid gland pathology

ANSWERS: 1D, 2B, 3G, 4C

An 85-year-old woman is brought to A&E from a nursing home with diffuse painful enlargement of the right parotid gland. Observations reveal a low-grade pyrexia.

D   Sialedenitis usually occurs due to bacterial infection from flora in the mouth. Factors impairing the drainage of saliva within the parotid duct are risk factors for infection e.g. dehydration, presence of a stone. There is often generalized diffuse enlargement of the gland and there may be overlying erythema or a low-grade pyrexia. Treatment involves the use of parotid massage and sialagogues to improve salivary flow and antibiotics to treat infection. If infection is not treated adequately there may be abscess formation which requires aspiration/surgical intervention.

A 28-year-old man presents with a discrete smooth firm 1.5 cm swelling over the tail of the right parotid gland. He feels that it has grown very slightly over the past 2 years. Fine needle aspiration reveals a mixture of epithelial, myoepithelial and stromal components.

B   Pleomorphic adenoma is the most common benign tumour of the parotid gland. It usually presents as a small slow-growing painless lump in the parotid gland. Diagnosis is achieved by fine needle aspiration. As the tumour is likely to grow albeit slowly and there is a very small risk of malignant transformation with time the treatment of choice is surgical excision via parotidectomy.

A 38-year-old woman with a history of rheumatoid arthritis complains of persistently dry mouth and eyes.

G   Sjogren's syndrome refers to an autoimmune disease that affects the exocrine glands that produce tears and saliva. It may occur as the primary pathology or may be secondary and associated with other autoimmune disease e.g. rheumatoid arthritis, SLE. Symptoms include dry mouth (xerostomia) and dry eyes (xerophthalmia). Schirmer's test may confirm significant pathological reduction in tear production. Ultrasound examination of the parotid glands may show typical multiple hypoechoic lesions that represent the lymphocytic infiltrates of the disease process. Blood tests may show the presence of anti-Ro or anti-La antibodies. A sub-labial (lip) biopsy to obtain definitive histology is often required to make a definitive diagnosis. Treatment is generally supportive with the use of artificial tears and saliva.

A 95-year-old man presents with a necrotic swelling over the right cheek which is fungating through the skin.

C   Primary squamous cell carcinoma of the parotid gland is rare and parotid SCC is usually metastatic from another source in the head and neck, e.g. cutaneous malignancy of the face and scalp. There may be a facial nerve palsy from infiltration of the facial nerve. Treatment may take the form of surgery, radiotherapy or both.

71 Complications of ENT surgery

ANSWERS: 1B, 2I, 3G, 4F

A 45-year-old woman complains of tongue numbness following excision of the right submandibular gland.

B   There are several nerves in close proximity to the submandibular gland which may be inadvertently injured during surgery. The lingual nerve loops close to the anterior portion of the gland where it gives off nerve roots extending into the submandibular ganglion. Injury may result in loss of sensation over the lateral aspect of the tongue. The hypoglossal nerve is at risk as it courses along the floor of the submandibular triangle. Injury will result in weakness of the muscles on one side of the tongue. Injury to the marginal mandibular branch of the facial nerve is also a recognized complication of surgery and results in a weakness of the muscles around the corner of the mouth with a resultant drooping of the lip on one side. It is not unusual for there to be a temporary neuropraxia of this nerve due to bruising from excessive intraoperative retraction. This may resolve over a period ranging from days to months.

A 34-year-old woman complains of sweating over her cheek when she eats following surgery to remove a neck lump.

I   Sweating associated with eating is called gustatory sweating. This is the classic feature of Frey's syndrome which is a complication of parotid gland surgery. The exact aetiology is not completely understood. It is hypothesized that there is division of the sympathetic fibres to the sweat glands and parasympathetic fibres to the parotid gland during surgery. These fibres are suggested to reinnervate abnormally in the postoperative period.

A 46-year-old patient reports profuse constant watery discharge from the left nostril following endoscopic sinus surgery.

G   CSF leak is a recognized complication of sinus surgery if there is inadvertent injury to the cribriform plate of the anterior skull base. It usually presents as persistent clear, watery rhinorrhoea. The patient is advised to collect a sample of the discharge which can be tested for beta-2-transferrin which is highly sensitive and specific for the presence of CSF. There is a risk of meningitis due to ascending infection which is estimated at around 10 per cent in the first few weeks after injury. Many leaks will settle conservatively but a persistent leak will require surgical repair.

A 36-year-old patient complains of crusting and recurrent minor nose bleeds about a year after septal surgery.

F   Septal perforation is a recognized complication of septoplasty surgery. In many cases particularly where the perforation lies posteriorly the patient has no symptoms. However, persistent perforations can be associated with crusting and bleeding. Often these symptoms can be managed by the use of topical moisturizing agents or septal buttons but in refractory cases surgical closure may be indicated.

72 Congenital causes of deafness

ANSWERS: 1K, 2I, 3G, 4E

An 8-year-old girl with profound sensorineural deafness and a goitre.

K   Pendred syndrome is an autosomal recessive genetic disorder characterized by bilateral sensorineural hearing loss and a goitre. Hypothyroidism may develop in some cases. MRI often reveals widened vestibular aqueducts or abnormalities of the inner ear e.g. Mondini dysplasia.

A 3-year-old boy with hearing loss, craniostenosis, exophthalmos and a parrot beak nose.

I   Crouzon syndrome is inherited in an autosomal dominant fashion. It is caused by aberrant fusion of the skull and facial bones during development. There is disruption of normal bone growth. On examination the most obvious features are the short and broad head caused by the cranial synostosis and low-set ears. Hearing impairment may be caused by abnormalities of the external canal or middle ear.

A 10-year-old with haematuria and bilateral sensorineural hearing loss. There is a history of nephritis in the family.

H   Alport syndrome is a genetic disorder which is usually inherited in an X-linked pattern although it may also be inherited in an autosomal recessive fashion. The gene mutation prevents the correct formation of type IV collagen which is an important structural component, particularly in the ear and kidney. The hearing loss typically develops gradually rather than presenting in infancy like many congenital hearing disorders. Treatment involves careful medical management of the renal disease as there is no known cure. The use of gene therapy is being explored as a possible therapeutic measure.

A 5-year-old boy with sensorineural hearing loss and syncopal episodes during stress.

E   Jervell and Lange-Nielsen syndrome is an autosomal recessive disorder caused by mutation in the *KCNE1* and *KCNQ1* genes. The mutation causes disruption of potassium channels that are present in the heart and inner ear. The prolonged QT interval may give rise to episodes of torsades de pointes, ventricular tachycardia and even ventricular fibrillation. There may be a history of syncopal episodes during stress or fright.

SECTION 6: OPHTHALMOLOGY

QUESTIONS

73 Red eye

A	scleritis	H	endophthalmitis
B	acute anterior uveitis	I	cicatricial pemphigoid
C	episcleritis	J	Stevens–Johnson syndrome
D	subtarsal foreign body	K	chronic blepharitis
E	atopic conjunctivitis	L	acute angle closure glaucoma
F	posterior uveitis	M	rosacea keratitis
G	conjunctival haemorrhage		

For each clinical scenario below give the most likely cause for the clinical findings. Each option may be used only once.

1   A 72-year-old man had cataract surgery about a week ago and developed a painful, red, congested eye, discharge, hypopyon and reduced red reflex. There was no fundus view.

2   A 25-year-old man presents with cold sores, oral ulcers, sore throat, myalgia, bilateral eyelid swelling and conjunctivitis with pseudomembranes.

3   An 8-year-old boy with eczema presents with photophobia, itching, stringy discharge, crusting of the eyelids, corneal ulcer and conjunctivitis.

4   A 45-year-old hyperopic woman presents to A&E with reduced vision to hand movements, painful left eye, frontal headache, vomiting, fixed mid-dilated pupil and a raised intraocular pressure of 50 mmHg.

Answers: see page 187

74 Diseases causing cataracts

A	homocystinuria	H	Wilson's disease
B	Marfan syndrome	I	Alport syndrome
C	Turner syndrome	J	myotonic dystrophy
D	Down syndrome	K	type II diabetes mellitus
E	syphilis	L	pemphigus
F	type I diabetes mellitus	M	Lowe syndrome
G	galactosaemia		

For each clinical scenario below give the most likely cause for the clinical findings. Each option may be used only once.

1   A child aged 5 years presents to the eye clinic with learning difficulties, bilateral cataracts, epicanthic folds, myopia, Brushfield spots and blue dot cataracts.

2   A 40-year-old man presents with frontal balding, muscle wasting, pigmentary retinopathy and Christmas tree cataracts.

3   A 57-year-old man presents to A&E with confusion, hepatosplenomegaly, hand tremor and green sunflower cataracts.

4   A 3-year-old child presents with learning difficulties and failure to thrive. She is found to have non-glucose reducing substance in the urine.

Answers: see page 188

75 Neuro-ophthalmology: pupils

A	tonic (Adie)	G	central Horner's syndrome
B	Marcus Gunn	H	traumatic mydriasis
C	III nerve palsy	I	Parinaud syndrome
D	Argyll Robertson	J	physiological anisocoria
E	preganglionic Horner's syndrome	K	senile miosis
F	postganglionic Horner's syndrome	L	aberrant III nerve regeneration
		M	pontine haemorrhage

For each clinical scenario below give the most likely cause for the clinical findings. Each option may be used only once.

1 A 50-year-old smoker presents with left-sided miosis, ptosis and anhydrosis. Chest x-ray shows an apical opacity in the left upper lobe. After testing with cocaine 4 per cent and adrenaline 1:1000, the left pupil remains undilated.

2 A 35-year-old myopic woman presents with a 2-day history of flashing lights, floaters, and a shadow across the right eye. The vision is reduced to 6/18 corrected and pupil testing shows an abnormal swinging light reflex. She is diagnosed with a right-sided retinal detachment.

3 A 52-year-old diabetic man presents to A&E with confusion, blurred vision, photophobia, headache, dizziness and bilaterally small irregular pupils. Blood tests are positive for VDRL.

4 A 45-year-old woman presents with sudden-onset blurred vision in the right eye of 6/12 with fixed dilated pupil, right-sided ptosis, and down-and-out looking right eye. She is hypertensive at 200/115 mmHg.

Answers: see page 189

76 Neuro-ophthalmology: visual fields

A   homonymous hemianopia   H   bitemporal hemianopia
B   superior quadrantanopia   I   arcuate scotoma
C   inferior quadrantanopia   J   centrocaecal scotoma
D   central scotoma   K   wedge scotoma
E   tunnel vision   L   nasal step
F   junctional scotoma   M   Seidel scotoma
G   altitudinal field defect

For each clinical scenario below give the most likely cause for the clinical findings. Each option may be used only once.

1   A 52-year-old man with night blindness presents to the eye clinic. Fundus examination shows spicule pigmentation, pale optic discs and arteriolar narrowing. Visual field testing shows bilateral symmetrical constricted fields.

2   A 34-year-old woman presents with decreased vision in the right eye to 6/18. She also complains of photophobia and pain on ocular movements. On examination she has a relative afferent pupillary defect, impaired colour vision and disc swelling. She has been diagnosed with multiple sclerosis a year previously. Visual field testing shows absent central field in the right eye.

3   A 75-year-old patient who has recently suffered a stroke complains of reduced vision to 6/24. Visual field testing shows a left hemi-field loss in both eyes.

4   A 55-year-old tall acromegalic man presents with symptoms of headache, diplopia and seesaw nystagmus. On examination there is bilateral papilloedema and retinopathy. Visual field testing shows bilateral symmetrical outer hemi-field loss.

Answers: see page 190

77 Ocular pharmacology

A   adrenaline 1 per cent

B   phenylephrine 10 per cent

C   cocaine 4 per cent

D   timolol maleate 0.5 per cent

E   apraclonidine 1 per cent

F   pilocarpine 4 per cent

G   atropine 1 per cent

H   dorzolamide 2 per cent

I   acetazolamide

J   mannitol

K   edrophonium

L   fluorescein 2 per cent

M   sodium cromoglicate 2 per cent

For each scenario below, suggest the most appropriate drug. Each option may be used only once.

1   A 32-year-old man was poked in the right eye by a branch. A few hours later he presents to A&E with a painful, photophobic left eye and reduced visual acuity of 6/60. A casualty officer applies a topical drop to diagnose a corneal abrasion.

2   A 30-year-old woman with presumed myasthenia gravis presents with bilateral ptosis, diplopia, variable ocular movements and increasing fatigability on exercise. She is injected with a drug as part of a Tensilon test. This improves the ptosis and diplopia after 5 minutes.

3   A 50-year-old man receives first-line topical therapy for reversing an acute angle closure glaucoma attack.

4   A 42-year-old woman presenting with severe pain and loss of vision secondary to an acute angle closure glaucoma attack requires intravenous therapy to reduce raised intraocular pressure of 60 mmHg.

Answers: see page 191

78 Ocular motility and ptosis

A	Marcus Gunn jaw-winking	H	mechanical ptosis
B	III cranial nerve palsy	I	levator dehiscence
C	Horner's syndrome	J	myotonic dystrophy
D	blepharophimosis syndrome	K	aberrant III nerve regeneration
E	myasthenia gravis	L	plexiform neurofibroma
F	simple congenital ptosis	M	blepharochalasis syndrome
G	blow-out fracture		

For each clinical scenario below give the most likely cause for the clinical findings. Each option may be used only once.

1   A 28-year-old man presents following an alleged assault. He has periorbital swelling and bruising with right-sided ptosis and enophthalmos. On examination there is restriction of up gaze and numbness of the right cheek.

2   A 40-year-old hypothyroid woman presents with bilateral asymmetrical ptosis, increasing on fatigability, with vertical diplopia and abnormal eye movements. The ptosis is relieved with ice packs.

3   A 70-year-old woman presents with bilateral symmetrical ptosis, with good levator function and high upper eyelid crease.

4   A 31-year-old man presents to his GP following sudden-onset ptosis associated with right-sided cluster headaches. On examination there is watering of the right eye, and a constricted right pupil with normal direct and consensual pupillary reflexes.

Answers: see page 192

79 Ocular and orbital pathology

A	basal cell carcinoma	H	thyroid eye disease
B	squamous cell carcinoma	I	lacrimal gland adenoma
C	sebaceous gland carcinoma	J	lymphoma
D	melanoma	K	carotid–cavernous fistula
E	Merkel cell carcinoma	L	orbital cellulitus
F	retinoblastoma	M	Wegener's granulomatosis
G	rhabdomyosarcoma			

For each clinical scenario below give the most likely cause for the clinical findings. Each option may be used only once.

1   An 8-year-old febrile child presents with swelling, ptosis and redness of the right eyelids. There is warmth of the overlying skin.

2   A 32-year-old woman presents with grittiness, photophobia, painful proptosis, lid swelling, periorbital oedema and chemosis. On examination there is presence of lid retraction, restriction of eye movements and raised intraocular pressure.

3   A 75-year-old man presents with a nodular blue-black lesion on the left upper eyelid. Two years ago he had an excised black pigmented conjunctival lesion found to be malignant. On this examination there is thickening of the eyelid margin and loss of eyelashes. Lid biopsy histology shows atypical melanocytes throughout the skin epidermis.

4   A 36-year-old man presents with a painful, proptosed left eye. He was involved in a road traffic accident a month previously. Since then he has complained of flushing noises in his head. On examination he has dilated conjunctival and episcleral vessels, raised intraocular pressure of 38 mmHg and left VI nerve palsy. He was referred to the neurosurgeons for further management.

Answers: see page 193

80 Retinal pathology

A	central retinal vein occlusion	G	age-related macular degeneration
B	macular hole	H	retinopathy of prematurity
C	retinal detachment	I	sickle-cell retinopathy
D	central retinal artery occlusion	J	diabetic maculopathy
E	proliferative diabetic	K	Coat's disease
	retinopathy	L	Best's vitelliform dystrophy
F	hypertensive retinopathy	M	retinal artery macroaneurysm

For each clinical scenario below, suggest the most appropriate retinal pathology. Each option may be used only once.

1   A 58-year-old smoker presents with sudden painless loss of vision in the right eye. On examination there is a relative afferent pupillary defect, and fundoscopy shows tortuous venous dilatation, flame and dot haemorrhages, and cotton wool spots.

2   A 42-year old smoker presents with blurred vision in the right eye. On fundus examination there is arteriolar narrowing with flame-shaped haemorrhages, optic disc swelling, cotton wool spots and a macular star.

3   A 34-year-old myope presents with reduced vision in the left eye, with a 2-day history of floaters, flashing lights and shadow across the vision.

4   A 28-year-old pregnant woman in the first trimester, with type 1 diabetes mellitus, presents complaining of blurred vision. On examination there is presence of retinal haemorrhages, cotton wool spots, exudates and new vessels on the optic disc and retina.

Answers: see page 194

81 Optic nerve pathology

A	optic disc drusen	H	Bergmeister papillae
B	optic disc pit	I	opticociliary shunts
C	optic disc coloboma	J	optic atrophy
D	morning glory syndrome	K	tilted disc
E	papilloedema	L	optic disc hypoplasia
F	myelinated optic disc	M	optic disc cupping
G	optic hypertrophy		

For each clinical scenario below give the most likely cause for the clinical findings. Each option may be used only once.

1   A 7-year-old is sent by the paediatric team for ophthalmic review. They are concerned about bilateral disc swelling on direct ophthalmoscopy, and CT scan which shows radio-opaque opacities at the optic nerves. On examination, fundoscopy shows unclear disc margins.

2   A 25-year-old man diagnosed with multiple sclerosis presents with reduced visual acuity of 6/9. He previously had an episode of painful loss of vision in the right eye a year ago.

3   A 28-year-old Afro-Caribbean woman presents after referral from her optician. She has decreased vision in both eyes to 6/9, a history of haloes around lights, and raised intraocular pressures of 40 mmHg and 33 mmHg in the right and left eyes respectively. Fundoscopy shows a characteristic optic disc appearance of glaucoma.

4   A 32-year-old obese patient presents with blurring of vision and frontal headaches for 2 weeks. The visual acuities are found to be 6/12 in each eye, and gross field testing reveals enlarged blind spots.

Answers: see page 195

82 Inherited eye disease

A   ankylosing spondylitis   H   aniridia
B   retinoblastoma   I   retinitis pigmentosa
C   Behçet disease   J   choroideraemia
D   type I neurofibromatosis   K   Leber's hereditary optic neuritis
E   type II neurofibromatosis   L   homocystinuria
F   multiple sclerosis   M   ocular albinism
G   Marfan syndrome

For each clinical scenario below give the most likely cause for the clinical findings. Each option may be used only once.

1   A 19-year-old tall myopic man presents to the clinic with a 2-day history of flashing lights and floaters in the right eye with retinal detachment. The lens in either eye is found to be dislocated superotemporally.

2   A 2-year-old child is brought to clinic following referral by the GP, who incidentally found left-sided abnormal white pupillary reflex, whereas the right eye had a normal red pupillary reflex. Fundoscopy reveals a white 'cottage-cheese like' mass with superficial blood vessels. CT scan shows an opacity at the left optic nerve.

3   A 34-year-old man presents with a painful left eye. On examination he is noted to have many eyelid lumps as well as nodules on the iris of both eyes. The pressure is raised in the left eye to 35 mmHg, and there are multiple choroidal naevi on fundoscopy.

4   A 40-year-old profoundly deaf man is referred by his GP for 'poor vision especially in the dark'. On examination fundoscopy shows spicule pigmentation, arteriolar narrowing and optic disc pallor, and field tests reveal bilateral tunnel vision.

Answers: see page 196

ANSWERS

73 Red eye

ANSWERS: 1H, 2J, 3E, 4L

> A 72-year-old man had cataract surgery about a week ago and developed a painful, red, congested eye, discharge, hypopyon and reduced red reflex. There was no fundus view.

H   Endophthalmitis is a devastating infection causing a painful loss of vision after ocular surgery. It is mainly caused by lid commensal bacteria such as *Staphlycoccus epidermidis* (70 per cent). Clinical features include pain, decreased acuity, anterior chamber activity, hypopyon, fibrin, absent red reflex and vitritis.

> A 25-year-old man presents with cold sores, oral ulcers, sore throat, myalgia, bilateral eyelid swelling and conjunctivitis with pseudomembranes.

J   Stevens–Johnson syndrome is a type III hypersensitivity reaction precipitated by drugs such as sulphonamides, NSAIDs and anticonvulsants, or infection (e.g. herpes simplex). The characteristic skin lesions are erythema multiforme with mucous membrane ulceration and scarring. Eye manifestations include eyelid oedema and pseudomembranous or membranous conjunctivitis. General features include fever, arthralgia, sore throat and malaise.

> An 8-year-old boy with eczema presents with photophobia, itching, stringy discharge, crusting of the eyelids, corneal ulcer and conjunctivitis.

E   Atopic keratoconjunctivitis is a chronic bilateral allergic ocular inflammation. It occurs mainly in childhood or early adult life especially in patients with atopic dermatitis. Clinical features consist of irritation, itching, stringy discharge, blepharitis, corneal pannus, conjunctival shortening and symblepharon. A differential of this condition could be vernal keratoconjunctivitis, which also occurs mainly in childhood and has a family history of atopy. Other features of this condition include the presence of Trantas' spots, cobblestone papillae and shield-shaped ulcers.

> A 45-year-old hyperopic woman presents to A&E with reduced vision to hand movements, painful left eye, frontal headache, vomiting, fixed mid-dilated pupil and a raised intraocular pressure of 50 mmHg.

L   Acute angle closure glaucoma is caused by the sudden closure of the angle. It mainly occurs in people aged over 40 years, with an increased incidence in the oriental/Asian population. Clinical features include sharp pain, decreased acuity, coloured haloes, nausea and vomiting. Examination reveals raised intraocular pressure of 50–100 mmHg, shallow anterior chamber, fixed mid-dilated pupil, ciliary injection, corneal oedema and anterior chamber inflammation.

74 Diseases causing cataracts

ANSWERS: 1D, 2J, 3H, 4G

A child aged 5 years presents to the eye clinic with learning difficulties, bilateral cataracts, epicanthic folds, myopia, Brushfield spots and blue dot cataracts.

D   Blue dot is the classic cataract found in patients with Down syndrome (chromosomal defect: trisomy 21). Other ocular features include strabismus, keratoconus, iris hypoplasia and unusual disc vasculature.

A 40-year-old man presents with frontal balding, muscle wasting, pigmentary retinopathy and Christmas tree cataracts.

J   Christmas tree cataract is a presenile cataract found in myotonic dystrophy. Other ocular features include ptosis, ophthalmoplegia, pupillary light-near dissociation and low intraocular pressure.

A 57-year-old man presents to A&E with confusion, hepatosplenomegaly, hand tremor and green sunflower cataracts.

H   Green sunflower cataract is found in patients with Wilson's disease (hepatolenticular degeneration). There is a deficiency in $a2$-globulin (caeruloplasmin) which results in copper deposition throughout the body. Other ocular features include Kayser-Fleischer ring (copper deposition in Desçemet's membrane) in the cornea, and accommodation problems.

A 3-year-old child presents with learning difficulties and failure to thrive. She is found to have a non-glucose reducing substance in the urine.

G   'Oil droplet' cataract is classically found in type II galactosaemia. It is an inborn error of metabolism, and is caused by the absence of galactose-1-phosphate uridyl transferase which results in an accumulation of galactose-1-phosphate. Affected children suffer from a failure to thrive. Other clinical features include psychomotor retardation, jaundice, diarrhoea, vomiting, renal disease and hepatosplenomegaly.

75 Neuro-ophthalmology: pupils

ANSWERS: 1E, 2B, 3D, 4C

A 50-year-old smoker presents with left-sided miosis, ptosis and anhydrosis. Chest x-ray shows an apical opacity in the left upper lobe. After testing with cocaine 4 per cent and adrenaline 1:1000, the left pupil remains undilated.

E   Preganglionic Horner's (second-order neuron) syndrome can be caused by various aetiologies such as Pancoast's tumour, carotid and aortic aneurysms. See Table 75.1 for an explanation of various Horner tests.

Table 75.1 Tests for Horner's syndrome

Eyedrops	Preganglionic	Central	Postganglionic	Normal
Cocaine 4%	2	2	2	1
Hydroxyamphetamine 1%	1	1	2	1
Adrenaline 1:1000	2	2	1	2

1, dilatation; 2, no dilatation.

A 35-year-old myopic woman presents with a 2-day history of flashing lights, floaters, and a shadow across the right eye. The vision is reduced to 6/18 corrected and pupil testing shows an abnormal swinging light reflex. She is diagnosed with a right-sided retinal detachment.

B   Marcus Gunn pupil or relative afferent pupillary defect is caused by an incomplete ipsilateral optic nerve lesion or severe retinal disease. In this scenario the patient has a retinal detachment causing the abnormal pupillary response.

A 52-year-old diabetic man presents to A&E with confusion, blurred vision, photophobia, headache, dizziness and bilaterally small irregular pupils. Blood tests are positive for VDRL.

D   Argyll Robertson pupil is characterized by bilateral small irregular pupils. Causes include neurosyphilis, diabetes mellitus and encephalitis. There is presence of light-near dissociation and these pupils are often difficult to dilate.

A 45-year-old woman presents with sudden-onset blurred vision in the right eye of 6/12 with fixed dilated pupil, right-sided ptosis, and down- and out-looking right eye. She is hypertensive at 200/115 mmHg.

C   III nerve palsy pupil is dilated, fixed and in the 'down and out' position. On examination one should urgently rule out surgical causes (posterior communicating artery aneurysm) in a painful III nerve palsy. The main causes of a painless III nerve palsy are hypertension and diabetes mellitus.

76 Neurophthalmology: visual fields

ANSWERS: 1E, 2D, 3A, 4H

A 52-year-old man with night blindness presents to the eye clinic. Fundus examination shows spicule pigmentation, pale optic discs and arteriolar narrowing. Visual field testing shows bilateral symmetrical constricted fields.

E   Tunnel vision is most commonly found in end-stage glaucoma or, as in this case, retinitis pigmentosa (RP). The patient actually has a variant of RP called Refsum's disease which has autosomal recessive inheritance. Other main clinical features associated with this condition are polyneuropathy, cerebellar ataxia and cardiomyopathy.

A 34-year-old woman presents with decreased vision in the right eye to 6/18. She also complains of photophobia and pain on ocular movements. On examination she has a relative afferent pupillary defect, impaired colour vision and disc swelling. She has been diagnosed with multiple sclerosis a year previously. Visual field testing shows absent central field in the right eye.

D   Central scotoma caused by papillitis is one of the clinical presentations of an optic neuritis. One-third of patients with multiple sclerosis will present with optic neuritis and two-thirds will have optic neuritis in the course of the disease. Optic neuritis is essentially a demyelinating or inflammatory process affecting the optic nerve.

A 75-year-old patient who has recently suffered a stroke complains of reduced vision to 6/24. Visual field testing shows a left hemi-field loss in both eyes.

A   Homonymous hemianopia is most commonly caused by cerebrovascular accident (stroke). Other possible causes are tumours and post-traumatic pathology. The hemianopic pathology occurs retrochiasmally; the further posterior the lesion in the optic tract, the more congruous (symmetrical) the hemianopia.

A 55-year-old tall acromegalic man presents with symptoms of headache, diplopia and seesaw nystagmus. On examination there is presence of bilateral papilloedema and retinopathy. Visual field testing shows bilateral symmetrical outer hemi-field loss.

H   Bitemporal hemianopia is associated with acromegalic patients.
         Acromegaly is caused by a hypersecretion of growth hormone by
         a pituitary acidophil adenoma. The hemianopia classically starts
         superiorly. Other ocular features of acromegaly are angioid streaks and
         optic atrophy.

77 Ocular pharmacology

ANSWERS: 1L, 2K, 3F, 4I

A 32-year-old man was poked in the right eye by a branch. A few
hours later he presents to A&E with a painful, photophobic left eye
and reduced visual acuity of 6/60. A casualty officer applies a topical
drop to diagnose a corneal abrasion.

L   Fluorescein is a yellow–orange topical dye which stains any epithelial
         defect and the surrounding loosely adherent epithelium. Fluorescein is
         also used for applanation tonometry, Seidel's test for aqueous leakage,
         Jones's test for tear duct patency, hard contact lens fitting and ocular
         angiography.

A 30-year-old woman with presumed myasthenia gravis presents with bilateral ptosis, diplopia, variable ocular movements and
increasing fatigability on exercise. She is injected with a drug as
part of a Tensilon test. This improves the ptosis and diplopia after
5 minutes.

K   Edrophonium is a reversible cholinesterase inhibitor. Myasthenia gravis
         can be confirmed by carrying out an ice-pack test or Tensilon test
         which is more specific. Whilst doing a Tensilon test it is important to
         have resuscitation equipment available, and intravenous atropine to
         counteract cholinergic overreaction. Alternatively one can carry out
         serology for anticholinesterase antibodies.

A 50-year-old man receives first-line topical therapy for reversing
an acute angle closure glaucoma attack.

F   Pilocarpine is a direct muscarinic agonist, and is the first-line topical
         therapy for acute angle closure glaucoma. It causes decreased aqueous
         production and uveoscleral outflow. In an acute angle closure glaucoma
         attack, pilocarpine causes pupillary constriction which opens the angle
         by pulling the peripheral iris away from the trabeculum.

A 42-year-old woman presenting with severe pain and loss of vision
secondary to an acute angle closure glaucoma attack requires intravenous therapy to reduce raised intraocular pressure of 60 mmHg.

I   Acetazolamide is a systemic carbonic anhydrase inhibitor. Its other uses
         include the treatment of papilloedema caused by raised intracranial

pressure. Side-effects included paraesthesia, malaise and depression. It is also a known precipitant of Stevens–Johnson syndrome.

78 Ocular motility and ptosis

ANSWERS: 1G, 2E, 3I, 4C

A 28-year-old man presents following an alleged assault. He has periorbital swelling and bruising with right-sided ptosis and enophthalmos. On examination there is restriction of up gaze and numbness of the right cheek.

G   Blow-out orbital floor fracture can be caused by a sudden increase in orbital pressure by any implement greater than 5 cm, such as a cricket ball or punching fist. Signs can include subconjuctival haemorrhage, periorbital haematoma and swelling, infraorbital anaesthesia, enophthalmos and diplopia on up gaze and down gaze. When a blow-out fracture is 'pure' it does not involve the orbital rim whereas the 'impure' form involves the orbital rim and facial bones.

A 40-year-old hypothyroid woman presents with bilateral asymmetrical ptosis, increasing on fatigability, with vertical diplopia and abnormal eye movements. The ptosis is relieved with ice packs.

E   Myasthenia gravis is an autoimmune disease characterized by fatigability and weakness of voluntary muscles. Weakness of the levator palpebrae superioris and extraocular muscles give rise to ptosis and diplopia. Other clinical features associated with myasthenia gravis include dysarthria, dysphagia and respiratory failure.

A 70-year-old woman presents with bilateral symmetrical ptosis, with good levator function and high upper eyelid crease.

I   Levator dehiscence occurs in the elderly due to stretching or disinsertion of the levator aponeurosis. The patient usually retains good levator function and presence of deep eyelid furrows due to high eyelid skin crease.

A 31-year-old man presents to his GP following sudden-onset ptosis associated with right-sided cluster headaches. On examination there is watering of the right eye, and a constricted right pupil with normal direct and consensual pupillary reflexes.

C   Horner's syndrome is caused by an oculosympathetic palsy. There are three subgroups of Horner's depending on the level of sympathetic chain being affected. The subgroups are central (first-order neuron), preganglionic (second-order neuron) and postganglionic (third-order neuron). This patient has a postganglionic Horner's. Common causes for this type are cluster headaches, internal carotid artery dissection, nasopharyngeal tumours, otitis media or cavernous sinus blockage.

The pupil anisocoria (difference in pupil sizes) is worse in the dark, hence the small constricted (myotic) pupil is more obvious in the dark.

79 Ocular and orbital pathology

ANSWERS: 1L, 2H, 3D, 4K

An 8-year-old febrile child presents with swelling, ptosis and redness of the right eyelids. There is warmth of the overlying skin.

L   Orbital cellulitis is a life-threatening infection of the soft tissues behind the orbital septum. It is usually caused by infection with *Streptococcus pneumoniae* or *S. pyogenes*, *Staphlococcus aureus* or *Haemophilus influenzae*. The initial infection can arise from sinusitis, local spread from dacryocystitis, preseptal cellulitis and dental infection. The patient presents with fever, swelling, erythema, proptosis around the eye, painful eye movements and optic nerve abnormalities. It is important to treat promptly with systemic intravenous antibiotics, and to monitor visual acuity and colour vision on a daily basis for any signs of deterioration.

A 32-year-old woman presents with grittiness, photophobia, painful proptosis, lid swelling, periorbital oedema and chemosis. On examination there is presence of lid retraction, restriction of eye movements and raised intraocular pressure.

H   Thyroid eye disease is an autoimmune condition in which IgG produces an increase in intraorbital fat and hypertrophy of extraocular muscles. Clinical features include soft tissue involvement, lid retraction, proptosis, optic neuropathy and restrictive myopathy. Severe disease may have to be treated by systemic steroids, extraocular muscle recession surgery, orbital decompression surgery and radiotherapy with or without immunosuppression.

A 75-year-old man presents with a nodular blue-black lesion on the left upper eyelid. Two years ago he had an excised black pigmented conjunctival lesion found to be malignant. On this examination there is thickening of the eyelid margin and loss of eyelashes. Lid biopsy histology shows atypical melanocytes throughout the skin epidermis.

D   Ocular melanoma is the most common ocular cancer, but is still rare. It accounts for 1 per cent of all eyelid tumours. Melanoma can start in the eyeball (95 per cent choroidal and 5 per cent iris), eyelid and conjunctiva. The three forms of eyelid melanoma are lentigo maligna, lentigo maligna melanoma and nodular melanoma (most common, as in this case). Treatment involves wide local excision by frozen section according to Breslow thickness. Adjunct therapy includes cryotherapy, radiotherapy and immunotherapy.

A 36-year-old man presents with a painful proptosed left eye. He was involved in a road traffic accident a month previously. Since then he has complained of flushing noises in his head. On examination he has dilated conjunctival and episcleral vessels, raised intraocular pressure of 38 mmHg and left VI nerve palsy. He was referred to the neurosurgeons for further management.

K   Carotid–cavernous fistula can be direct or indirect. This case is an example of a direct carotid–cavernous fistula. Investigation is by arterial angiography and treatment involves interventional radiology with a detachable balloon occlusion of the fistula.

80 Retinal pathology

ANSWERS: 1A, 2F, 3C, 4E

A 58-year-old smoker presents with sudden painless loss of vision in the right eye. On examination there is a relative afferent pupillary defect, and fundoscopy shows tortuous venous dilatation, flame and dot haemorrhages, and cotton wool spots.

A   Central retinal vein occlusion can be of two types, non-ischaemic or ischaemic, and is mainly caused by hypertension and diabetes mellitus. It is one of the commonest causes of sudden unilateral blurred vision. The visual acuity ranges from 6/36 to counting fingers and there is usually presence of an afferent pupillary defect. Clinical features include venous tortuosity, dot-blot and flame-shaped haemorrhages, cotton wool spots and disc oedema on fundoscopy. Complications include rubeotic glaucoma due to ischaemia of the retina. This needs to be treated with panretinal photocoagulation.

A 42-year-old smoker presents with blurred vision in the right eye. On fundus examination there is arteriolar narrowing with flame-shaped haemorrhages, optic disc swelling, cotton wool spots and a macular star.

F   Hypertensive retinopathy can be graded 1 to 4. Clinical features include an arteriosclerosis of varying severity. The main causes are essential hypertension, renal disease, endocrine disease such as Cushing's, eclampsia and coarctation of the aorta. Complications of hypertension include left ventricular failure, renal failure, strokes, hypertensive encephalopathy, myocardial infarction and retinopathy.

A 34-year-old myope presents with reduced vision in the left eye, with a 2-day history of floaters, flashing lights and shadow across the vision.

C   Retinal detachment (RD) is a separation of the sensory retina from the retinal pigment epithelium (RPE) by subretinal fluid (SRF). There are two types of retinal detachment, rhegmatogenous and non-rhegmatogenous. A rhegmatogenous RD is due to a full-thickness defect in the sensory retina which allows SRF derived from the vitreous into the subretinal space. The non-rhegmatogenous RD can be caused by two mechanisms. The first involves traction between vitreoretinal membranes pulling the sensory retina away from the RPE. The other mechanism is exudative where the SRF derived from retinal blood supply is transmitted to the SRF through the damaged RPE.

A 28-year-old pregnant woman in the first trimester, with type 1 diabetes mellitus, presents complaining of blurred vision. On examination there is presence of retinal haemorrhages, cotton wool spots, exudates and new vessels on the optic disc and retina.

E   Proliferative diabetic retinopathy is considered to be end-stage diabetic retinopathy. Pregnancy can rapidly increase the progression of even mild retinopathy in a short time. This patient will have to undergo bilateral laser panretinal photocoagualation to treat this sight-threatening condition.

81 Optic nerve pathology

ANSWERS: 1A, 2J, 3M, 4E

A 7-year-old is sent by the paediatric team for ophthalmic review. They are concerned about bilateral disc swelling on direct ophthalmoscopy, and CT scan which shows radio-opaque opacities at the optic nerves. On examination, fundoscopy shows unclear disc margins.

A   Optic nerve drusen is a congenital condition and is often familial. It is bilateral in 70 per cent. The drusen consists of hyaline-like calcific material. It gives the appearance of elevated discs in buried drusen cases, and autofluorescence on fluorescein angiography. It can be diagnosed on ultrasound and CT scan. Drusen can cause various complications such as visual field defects and peripapillary choroidal neovascularization. It is associated with retinitis pigmentosa, angioid streaks and vitreous haemorrhage.

A 25-year-old man diagnosed with multiple sclerosis presents with reduced visual acuity of 6/9. He previously had an episode of painful loss of vision in the right eye a year ago.

J   Optic atrophy can be caused by congenital or hereditary causes such as Leber's hereditary optic atrophy. Other causes are secondary to raised intracranial pressure, retinal disease, optic neuritis or neuropathy, optic nerve compression, trauma and secondary to metabolic disease.

A 28-year-old Afro-Caribbean woman presents after referral from her optician. She has decreased vision in both eyes to 6/9, a history of haloes around lights, and raised intraocular pressures of 40 mmHg and 33 mmHg in the right and left eyes respectively. Fundoscopy shows a characteristic optic disc appearance of glaucoma.

M   Optic disc cupping is a characteristic feature of glaucomatous nerve fibre damage. The visual loss may occur by direct mechanical effect on the nerve fibres, vascular insufficiency to the optic nerve head and ganglion cell death.

A 32-year-old obese patient presents with blurring of vision and frontal headaches for 2 weeks. The visual acuities are found to be 6/12 in each eye, and gross field testing reveals enlarged blind spots.

E   Papilloedema is swelling of the optic nerve head due to raised intracranial pressure. It is believed that raised intracranial CSF pressure around the optic nerve results in transudation of fluid into the nerve with obstruction of axoplasmic transport. It is the intra-axonal swelling of the axons with accumulation of mitochondria that causes the initial disc swelling. Treatment involves systemic acetazolamide. In severe cases, neurosurgery is required in the form of a ventriculoperitoneal shunt.

82 Inherited eye disease

ANSWERS: 1G, 2B, 3D, 4I

A 19-year-old tall myopic man presents to the clinic with a 2-day history of flashing lights and floaters in the right eye with retinal detachment. The lens in either eye is found to be dislocated super-otemporally.

G   Marfan syndrome is an autosomal dominant condition associated with a defect in fibrillin synthesis (defect at chromosome 15). There is an increased risk of associated cardiovascular complications including dissecting aortic aneurysms and aortic regurgitation. Ocular features include bilateral superotemporal subluxation, microspherophakia, flat and enlarged cornea, myopia, retinal detachment, angle anomalies and glaucoma.

A 2-year-old child is brought to clinic following referral by the GP, who incidently found left-sided abnormal white pupillary reflex, whereas the right eye had a normal red pupillary reflex. Fundoscopy reveals a white 'cottage-cheese like' mass with superficial blood vessels. CT scan shows an opacity at the left optic nerve.

B   Retinoblastoma is the most common primary intraocular malignancy in childhood. It can present in two forms, endophytic and exophytic. The inheritance is sporadic in 60 per cent and hereditary in 40 per cent; the defect is at 13q14. This presents within 2 years of life and is associated with strabismus in 20 per cent of cases. Other associated clinical features are secondary glaucoma, proptosis, lymph node metastasis and raised intracranial pressure.

Treatment consists of transpupillary thermotherapy, brachytherapy, cryotherapy, enucleation and chemotherapy depending on the size of the tumour.

A 34-year-old man presents with a painful left eye. On examination he is noted to have many eyelid lumps as well as nodules on the iris of both eyes. The pressure is raised in the left eye to 35 mmHg, and there are multiple choroidal naevi on fundoscopy.

D   Type 1 neurofibromatosis is an autosomal dominant condition; the gene defect is at 17q11. Clinical features that may be seen in this disorder are orbital gliomas, eyelid neurofibromas, iris Lisch nodules, glaucoma and fundal lesions such as choroidal naevi and retinal astrocytomas.

A 40-year-old profoundly deaf man is referred by his GP for 'poor vision especially in the dark'. On examination fundoscopy shows spicule pigmentation, arteriolar narrowing and optic disc pallor, and field tests reveal bilateral tunnel vision.

I   Retinitis pigmentosa is a diffuse retinal dystrophy which affects the rod system. There is a variety of inheritance mechanisms such as sporadic, autosomal dominant/recessive and X-linked recessive. It commonly presents in the third decade. Investigations (e.g. electroretinogram) show a reduced scotopic rod response. Visual fields show tunnel vision. There are other systemic associations of retinitis pigmentosa such as Usher syndrome, as in this case.

SECTION 7: ANAESTHESIA AND CRITICAL CARE

QUESTIONS

83 Arterial blood gases

Which of the blood gases in Table 83.1 best fits the following scenarios?

Table 83.1 Arterial blood gases

	A	B	C	D	E	F	G	H	I	J
pH	7.0	7.35	7.0	7.41	7.35	7.5	7.25	7.55	7.39	7.4
PaO_2 (kPa)	12.2	10.5	5.5	12.5	7.8	14	9.4	10.5	11.9	12.4
$PaCO_2$ (kPa)	2.2	4.4	8.0	4.6	4.5	2.9	8.9	6.0	5.4	3.9
HCO_3^- (mmol/L)	15	23	18	26	23	23	22	48	25	23

1   A 69-year-old male patient on the cardiac ward collapses. He has no pulse and cardiopulmonary resuscitation is initiated. ECG shows ventricular fibrillation. His condition deteriorates as he shows asystole after 10 minutes of resuscitation. An arterial blood gas sample is taken during resuscitation while the patient is being ventilated with a bag and mask.

2   A 20-year-old man presents semiconscious to A&E. He is known to have a family history of insulin-dependent diabetes. He takes deep breaths and his breath smells ketotic.

3   A 32-year-old woman is brought to A&E by ambulance from a shopping centre. She complains of acute onset of shortness of breath and atypical chest pain. On examination she is tachypnoeic, anxious and has carpopedal spasm.

4   You are called to the ward at 1 a.m. to see a 79-year-old patient with breathing difficulties. He is an ex-smoker with COPD. On oxygen at 4 L/min, pulse oximetry shows SaO_2 at 94 per cent. Respiratory rate is 30 breaths/min. On examination his hands feel warm and the anaesthetist notes that he has a poor cough.

5   A 25-year-old known asthmatic is complaining of difficulty breathing in A&E. She has been feeling unwell for some days. She is unable to speak a full sentence and her lips look cyanosed.

ANSWERS: see page 211

84 Airway management (i)

A oropharyngeal airway size 4
B laryngeal mask airway size 4
C oral endotracheal tube cuffed
   size 8
D Magill forceps
E reinforced cuffed endotracheal
   tube

F nasopharyngeal airway
G laryngeal mask airway size 2
H oral endotracheal tube uncuffed
   size 3.5
I fibreoptic laryngoscope
J bougie

For each of the scenarios below select the most appropriate piece of equipment to maintain the airway. Each option may be used only once.

1   A 20-year-old male needs an appendicectomy urgently. He is septic and unwell. The surgeon wants to operate as soon as possible.

2   A newborn baby has difficulty breathing and needs ventilation.

3   A 2-year-old child needs a circumcision under general anaesthesia.

4   A man with an unstable cervical spine fracture needs to be intubated safely.

5   An attempt at tracheal intubation is made on a 65-year-old man. Direct laryngoscopy reveals a view of the posterior arytenoids only and the endotracheal tube passes into the oesophagus.

ANSWERS: see page 212

85 Airway management (ii)

A   awake fibreoptic intubation
B   laryngeal mask ventilation
C   rapid sequence intubation

D   asleep fibreoptic intubation
E   cricothyroidotomy
F   gas induction of anaesthesia

For each of the scenarios below select the most appropriate anaesthetic
technique to secure or maintain the airway. Each option may be used only once.

1   A 4-year-old boy is admitted with acute epiglottitis and stridor, and is
    deteriorating.

2   A 70-year-old male is admitted for an emergency laparotomy for small bowel
    obstruction.

3   A 50-year-old female with a stridor collapses in the resus bay in the emergency
    department. Facemask ventilation with Guedel airway and 2-handed technique
    fails, and insertion of a laryngeal mask is unsuccessful. Attempts at tracheal
    intubation also fail. She becomes cyanotic and her pulse oximetry records 58
    per cent.

4   A 20-year-old male is admitted with Ludwig's angina and is drooling saliva and
    has severe trismus.

ANSWERS: see page 213

86 Intravenous access

A	24G cannula	F	Swan introducer (7F)
B	22G cannula	G	arterial cannulation line
C	14G cannula	H	Hickman line
D	intraosseous needle	I	pulmonary artery catheter
E	three-lumen central venous line	J	femoral line insertion

For each clinical scenario suggest the most appropriate means of intravenous access. Each option may be used only once.

1   A man is admitted to A&E after a road traffic accident. His blood pressure is 75/40 mmHg and heart rate 120/min. He complains of marked abdominal pain.

2   A 45-year-old woman has been diagnosed with metastatic breast cancer and requires repeated administration of intravenous chemotherapy. She has poor peripheral veins.

3   A baby is admitted with severe diarrhoea and needs urgent resuscitation as his consciousness level is deteriorating. The team is unable to find a vein to insert an intravenous cannula.

4   A patient is in ITU with septic shock. He needs access to deliver noradrenaline (norepinephrine) infusion to increase his blood pressure. He has a large cannula in the dorsum of the hand.

5   The anaesthetist would like intravenous access for the induction of anaesthesia in a fit and well adult.

ANSWERS: see page 214

87 Pain relief

A	paracetamol and dihydrocodeine	F	paracetamol
B	thoracic epidural analgesia	G	morphine sulphate SR
C	patient-controlled analgesia with ketorolac	H	lumbar epidural analgesia
D	paracetamol, diclofenac and immediate-release morphine	I	patient-controlled analgesia with morphine
E	fentanyl patch	J	paracetamol and diclofenac sodium

For each clinical scenario below select the most appropriate choice of pain relief. Each option may be used only once.

1 An 18-year-old man with a diagnosis of osteosarcoma has been admitted to the cardiothoracic unit for removal of a metastasis in his right upper lung lobe. He requires a thoracotomy.

2 A 70-year-old day surgery patient needs analgesia prescribing following unilateral varicose vein surgery. The only past medical history of note is occasional complaints of heartburn.

3 A 65-year-old man with colon cancer requires an anterior resection. He has a significant history of chronic obstructive airways disease treated with high-dose inhaled steroids and aminophylline. His peak expiratory flow rate is 195 mL/s. An ITU bed has been booked for his postoperative recovery.

4 A 45-year-old woman is undergoing a left-sided mastectomy for breast cancer. She is very anxious and particularly worried about her postoperative pain as, for previous wide-local excision surgery, she had to wait for her pain-relieving medication.

ANSWERS: see page 216

88 Drugs for anaesthesia

A	midazolam	F	suxamethonium
B	atracurium	G	lorazepam
C	tubocurare	H	ketamine
D	propofol	I	fentanyl
E	sevoflurane	J	cyclopropane

For each of the scenarios below select the most appropriate choice of drug. Each option may be used only once.

1   A 16-year-old male has been admitted to the A&E department with a diagnosis of acute appendicitis. The surgical team decides to proceed to appendicectomy immediately. After assessing the patient the anaesthetist plans to perform a rapid sequence intubation.

2   A 24-year-old woman is scheduled to undergo varicose vein surgery. She is a fit non-smoker and drinks 6 units of alcohol a week. Her last meal was 6 hours ago. The anaesthetist picks a drug for intravenous induction of anaesthesia.

3   A 6-year-old girl scheduled for a tonsillectomy is severely needle-phobic. It is felt that although an intravenous anaesthetic would be preferable, in this particular situation it would be too traumatic. After discussion with the mother and child, the anaesthetist has offered the choice of a 'gas induction'.

4   A 51-year-old woman is scheduled for a hysterectomy. The surgeons request muscle relaxation. She has been nil by mouth for 10 hours and has no risk of aspirating.

ANSWERS: see page 217

89 Oxygen therapy

A	nasal cannula	F	CPAP circuit
B	tracheal mask	G	28 per cent fixed-performance
C	non-rebreathe mask with		mask
	reservoir bag	H	nebulizer
D	endotracheal intubation	I	neonatal mask
E	Bain circuit	J	cold-water humidifier

For each clinical scenario below select the most appropriate choice of oxygen therapy. Each option may be used only once.

1   A 20-year-old man was been knocked from his motorbike. He has a clear and patent airway. Examination reveals a possible fractured pelvis and right femur.

2   A 65-year-old man with COPD was admitted to the ward with an infective exacerbation of COPD. Pulse oximetry shows 87 per cent oxygen saturation on air. He has a letter from his chest physician which he has been told to keep with him at all times. It describes that the patient relies on a hypoxic ventilatory drive.

3   A 67-year-old man develops shortness of breath, wheeze and is coughing up frothy red sputum. His oxygenation is deteriorating as he is transferred to ITU.

4   A 25-year-old woman is admitted to A&E with an acute exacerbation of her asthma. Examination reveals wheeze throughout both lung fields.

ANSWERS: see page 218

90 Preoperative investigation

A   chest x-ray
B   transfer factor
C   peak flow rate
D   pulmonary function tests
E   CT scan
F   ventilation–perfusion scan

G   echocardiography
H   ECG
I   body plethysmogram
J   MRI of chest
K   PET imaging

For each clinical scenario below suggest the most appropriate investigation. Each option may be used only once.

1   A 75-year-old man with a history of smoking 10–15 cigarettes a day for 35 years is admitted for elective major surgery. He has a productive cough.

2   A patient is scheduled for an anterior resection. He has COPD and complains that he has had more chest tightness recently. You wish to assess his lung function in the pre-assessment clinic.

3   A 75-year-old woman attends the pre-assessment clinic prior to total hip replacement. She has had episodes of shortness of breath, chest pain and syncope.

4   A patient is admitted for vascular surgery to improve the blood flow to his right leg. He is functionally severely compromised. He reports that he has started to get chest pains when he walks for over 30 yards.

ANSWERS: see page 220

91 Support in critical care

A	adrenaline (epinephrine)	F	intra-aortic balloon pump
B	noradrenaline (norepinephrine)	G	levosimendan
C	dopamine	H	intravenous fluid challenge
D	dopexamine	I	labetalol
E	vasopressin	J	glyceryl trinitrate (GTN)

For each clinical scenario below select the most appropriate choice of supportive measure or drug for intravenous infusion or bolus. Each option may be used only once.

1   A 58-year-old man presents with central chest pain radiating into his back. He has a heart rate 95/min, BP 170/95 mmHg and poor urine output. ECG is normal. He is awaiting a CT scan of his chest.

2   A 70-year-old diabetic Asian woman presents with intermittent central chest pain. She is on GTN, insulin and a heparin infusion in the cardiac unit. Coronary angiogram shows severe triple-vessel disease. She is awaiting a coronary artery bypass graft but presents with further chest pain in the night. Pulse 70/min, BP 90/50 mmHg, troponin T 0.05.

3   A 28-year-old male intravenous drug abuser is admitted to ITU with a red, inflamed mass in his groin. He is due to go to theatre to have the mass explored. Heart rate is 115/min, BP 80/30 mmHg, and he is oliguric.

4   A 35-year-old man with septic shock is being treated in ITU. His mean arterial blood pressure has dropped to 65 mmHg despite adequate fluid resuscitation.

5   An 8-year-old girl has a cardiopulmonary arrest following a bee sting.

ANSWERS: see page 221

92 Risk and side-effects of general anaesthesia

A	1 in 5	E	1 in 3000
B	1 in 50	F	1 in 10000
C	1 in 300	G	1 in 100000
D	1 in 1000	H	1 in 600000

For each of the scenarios below select the associated incidence. Each option may be used only once.

1   The risk of sore throat following an anaesthetic.

2   The risk of awareness during anaesthesia.

3   The risk of getting hepatitis B following a blood transfusion.

4   The risk of death during anaesthesia.

5   The risk of failed intubation in the obstetric population.

ANSWERS: see page 222

93 Anaphylaxis

A	remove potential allergen, call for help, maintain the airway and administer oxygen 100 per cent	D	1 in 1300
		E	1 in 13 000
		F	1 in 130 000
B	give 1 L of 0.9 per cent saline or Ringer's solution at high rate via an intravenous cannula of an appropriate gauge to treat hypotension	G	adrenaline 50 mcg (0.5 mL of 1:10 000 solution) intramuscularly
		H	adrenaline 50 mcg (0.5 mL of 1:10 000 solution) intravenously
C	remove potential allergen and give intravenous adrenaline (epinephrine) in small boluses as required by experienced doctor to treat hypotension, wheeze, bronchospasm and oedema.	I	adrenaline 50 mcg (5 mL of 1:10 000 solution) intravenously
		J	serum epinephrine levels
		K	serum IgE levels
		L	serum tryptase levels

For each question regarding anaphylaxis, give the most appropriate answer. Each option may be used only once.

1   A 20-year-old man is being given intravenous co-amoxiclav on the ward and has sudden-onset rash, urticaria, hypotension, wheeze, bronchospasm and oedema. What are your first steps in the management of this man?

2   What is the lifetime incidence of anaphylaxis in the UK population?

3   What is the appropriate dose of adrenaline (epinephrine) and its administration route for the treatment of life-threatening anaphylaxis?

4   What serum indicator is most useful in the diagnosis of anaphylaxis?

ANSWERS: see page 223

94 Anaesthetic emergencies

A	malignant hyperthermia	F	hypotension on induction
B	large pulmonary embolism	G	failure to intubate
C	anaphylaxis	H	bronchospasm
D	laryngospasm	I	oesophageal intubation
E	regurgitation and aspiration	J	incomplete reversal of paralysis

For each clinical scenario below give the most likely cause for the clinical findings. Each option may be used only once.

1 An obese 40-year-old woman undergoes examination under anaesthetic for an anal fissure. She is induced with propofol and alfentanil. Anaesthesia is maintained with isoflurane. She is lightly anaesthetized in a head-down position with a laryngeal mask airway in place and a clear airway. Ten minutes after the procedure has commenced, she develops marked stridor and reduction in tidal volumes.

2 A 40-year-old woman is undergoing emergency surgery for a comminuted tibial fracture. While the surgeon is manipulating the fracture, the anaesthetist notices a sudden loss of end tidal carbon dioxide trace.

3 A 24-year-old woman is undergoing a diagnostic laparoscopy. She has never had a general anaesthetic before. Following intravenous induction, anaesthesia is maintained with isoflurane. The patient develops a sudden tachycardia. A rapid increase in the end tidal carbon dioxide trace is noted.

4 A 70-year-old woman has difficulty breathing after extubation following a general anaesthetic for an umbilical hernia repair. She had been intubated and ventilated following 100 mg of propofol, 10 mg of vecuronium and 100 mcg of fentanyl. Anaesthesia was maintained with isoflurane and a further 4 mg of vecuronium was administered 15 minutes before extubation.

ANSWERS: see page 224

ANSWERS

83 Arterial blood gases

ANSWERS: 1C, 2A, 3F, 4G, 5E

A 69-year-old male patient on the cardiac ward collapses. He has no pulse and cardiopulmonary resuscitation is initiated. ECG shows ventricular fibrillation. His condition deteriorates as he shows asystole after 10 minutes of resuscitation. An arterial blood gas sample is taken during resuscitation while the patient is being ventilated with a bag and mask.

C   This patient has suffered a loss of cardiac output and ventilatory failure. He is being poorly ventilated during the resuscitation. An arterial blood gas sample would show a severe metabolic acidosis as a result of loss of cardiac output and poor tissue perfusion. Hypoxia and hypercarbia result from poor ventilation. Hypercarbia would worsen the acidosis. This results in combined respiratory and metabolic acidosis.

A 20-year-old man presents semiconscious to A&E. He is known to have a family history of insulin-dependent diabetes. He takes deep breaths and his breath smells ketotic.

A   Diabetic ketoacidosis can be the presenting feature of an undiagnosed young diabetic. It may be defined by serum bicarbonate < 16 mmol/L, ketonaemia, +/− hyperglycaemia, +/− mental impairment. His arterial blood gas would show a severe metabolic acidosis with a low carbon dioxide secondary to increased respiratory drive from the acidosis.

A 32-year-old woman is brought to A&E by ambulance from a shopping centre. She complains of acute onset of shortness of breath and atypical chest pain. On examination she is tachypnoeic, anxious and has carpopedal spasm.

F   This woman has a good history for a diagnosis of hyperventilation syndrome. Her arterial blood gases would reveal a respiratory alkalosis. Carpopedal spasm is caused by acute secondary hypocalcaemia as a result of the alkalosis.

You are called to the ward at 1 a.m. to see a 79-year-old patient with breathing difficulties. He is an ex-smoker with COPD. On oxygen at 4 L/min, pulse oximetry shows SaO_2 at 94 per cent. Respiratory rate is 30 breaths/min. On examination his hands feel warm and the anaesthetist notes that he has a poor cough.

G   This man with COPD probably maintains an oxygen saturation within the low 90s (per cent), so a lower oxygen saturation does not necessarily imply an acute hypoxia. It should be interpreted in the context of his baseline oxygen saturation. In this case the patient is tachypnoeic with a poor cough. He is warm and therefore vasodilated. This would fit a picture of exacerbation of type II respiratory failure ($PaO_2 < 8$ kPa and $pCO_2 > 6$ kPa) leading to a respiratory acidosis. The CO_2 retention is the cause of the vasodilated circulation.

A 25-year-old known asthmatic is complaining of difficulty breathing in A&E. She has been feeling unwell for some days. She is unable to speak a full sentence and her lips look cyanosed.

E   This girl is presenting with acute type I respiratory failure secondary to asthma. She is likely to have a normal or slightly low CO_2. One should be wary of the asthmatic patient whose CO_2 starts to rise as this implies that the patient is tiring and developing a ventilatory failure. This would be a clear indication for ITU/specialist care.

84 Airway management (i)

ANSWERS: 1C, 2H, 3G, 4I, 5J

Airway management during anaesthesia follows three principles:
- maintaining a clear airway
- protecting the airway from soiling by blood, secretions and gastric contents
- providing a secure and reliable airway.

Every patient should have the airway assessed on the preoperative visit. Risk factors for a difficult airway or of aspiration should be identified and a plan formulated for how the airway will be managed.

A 20-year-old male needs an appendicectomy urgently. He is septic and unwell. The surgeon wants to operate as soon as possible.

C   This patient needs a protected airway rapidly secured after induction of anaesthesia. He is at high risk of regurgitation and aspiration on induction. A rapid sequence induction should be performed and the airway protected with a cuffed endotracheal tube (ETT). Size 8–9 is appropriate for a male and size 7–8 would be appropriate for females.

A newborn baby has difficulty breathing and needs ventilation.

H   This baby needs tracheal intubation to protect the airway and to facilitate ventilation. Though laryngeal mask airways (LMA) have been used in resuscitations they would not be appropriate for prolonged ventilation. Uncuffed tracheal tubes are used in babies and children under the age of 7 years or body weight less than 35 kg. These reduce the incidence of post-extubation stridor and tracheal stenosis. There should be a noticeable air leak around the tube at an airway pressure of 25 cmH$_2$0. A newborn takes a size 3–3.5 tube, and after age 12 months tubes can be sized using the formula: ETT internal diameter (age/4) + 4 mm.

A 2-year-old child needs a circumcision under general anaesthesia.

G   Circumcision is an elective procedure so the child would be starved. It is unlikely that a healthy normal 2-year-old would be at risk of regurgitation, so it would be appropriate to use a LMA. These come in sizes 1, 2, 2.5, 3, 4 and 5. A size 2 is appropriate for ventilating children 6–20 kg.

A man with an unstable cervical spine fracture needs to be intubated safely.

I   In a patient with an unstable cervical spine fracture an awake fibreoptic intubation is indicated. This allows the airway to be secured without undue manipulation of the cervical spine.

An attempt at tracheal intubation is made on a 65-year-old man. Direct laryngoscopy reveals a view of the posterior arytenoids only and the endotracheal tube passes into the oesophagus.

J   Failure to intubate is not an emergency if the patient's airway can be maintained and protected and they can be adequately ventilated. A decision needs to be made to ascertain whether further attempts at intubation should be made or some other method of airway maintenance should be employed. In the event that further attempts at intubation are made, the patient's head position should be fully optimized and both appropriate adjunct equipment and senior help should be available. A gum elastic bougie solves many of the simpler failures to intubate.

85 Airway management (ii)

ANSWERS 1F, 2C, 3E, 4A

A 4-year-old boy is admitted with acute epiglottitis and stridor, and is deteriorating.

F   Acute epiglottis in children is a potentially life-threatening condition. The child is kept sitting and disturbing the child must be kept to a minimum (including attempts at insertion of an IV cannula or laryngoscopy). It may be a life-threatening airway emergency and induction of anaesthesia is by gas induction.

A 70-year-old male is admitted for an emergency laparotomy for small bowel obstruction.

C   The risk of aspiration (where acid and/or stomach contents are regurgitated and enters the lungs) in the general, a starved population is relatively rare and occurs 1 in 2000 to 1 in 3000. It occurs more frequently in patients with ASA III or IV status and in emergency cases (as high as 1 in 600). To minimize the risk, a rapid sequence induction (RSI) is performed i.e. induction of anaesthesia with thiopentone and a rapid-onset muscle relaxant to facilitate tracheal intubation. In addition, cricoid pressure is applied to the cricoid cartilage to compress the oesophagus to prevent aspiration of stomach contents.

A 50-year-old female with a stridor collapses in the resus bay in the emergency department. Facemask ventilation with Guedel airway and 2-handed technique fails, and insertion of a laryngeal mask is unsuccessful. Attempts at tracheal intubation also fail. She becomes cyanotic and her pulse oximetry records 58 per cent.

E   This is an airway emergency and repeated attempts at tracheal intubation must be avoided ('solution fixation'). This is a 'can't intubate, can't ventilate' scenario and requires an invasive technique to secure the airway. It involves puncturing the cricothyroid membrane and inserting an airway device for ventilation. These cricothyroidotomy devices come in various diameters (cricothyroidotomy cannula 2 mm, large cannula 4 mm and tracheostomy tubes > 6 mm). The diameter is dictated by the type of ventilation required, e.g. high-pressure jet ventilation or low-pressure ventilation.

A 20-year-old male is admitted with Ludwig's angina and has severe trismus.

A   Patients with an anticipated difficult airway and who are predicted to be difficult to ventilate after induction of anaesthesia are at risk of a 'can't intubate, can't ventilate' (CICV) scenario. Such patients should have an awake technique to secure their airway. In patients with non-obstructing upper airways, the gold standard of securing the airway is by using awake fibreoptic intubation. Those with an obstructing upper airway (e.g. epiglottis in adults or laryngeal cancer) may require an awake tracheostomy (this will need discussion and planning with senior and experienced anaesthetists and ENT/maxillofacial surgeons).

86 Intravenous access

ANSWERS: 1C, 2H, 3D, 4E, 5B

A man is admitted to A&E after a road traffic accident. His blood pressure is 75/40 mmHg and heart rate 120/min. He complains of marked abdominal pain.

C   Large-bore intravenous cannulation is urgently required in this patient. He has active intra-abdominal bleeding. According to trauma guidelines, two large-bore cannulae should be established and fluid resuscitation commenced.

The diameter of the cannula determines the infusion rate as flow is directly proportional to the radius to the power of 4. Therefore, if blood has to be given where larger particles such as erythrocytes are transfused, a larger bore cannula is preferred. In resuscitation, 14G cannulae are the intravenous access of choice, and two 14G should be inserted (flow rate of 250 mL/min). In exceptional circumstances such as liver surgery where major blood loss is expected a Swan introducer is used (7F).

Cannula gauges are defined by steel wire gauge. This is the number of steel wires of the same diameter as the cannula that fit into a standard sized hole. Therefore the higher the gauge number the smaller the cannula. Cannulae are colour-coded:

- yellow – 24G suitable for neonates and babies
- blue – 22G
- pink – 20G suitable for i.v. crystalloid
- green – 18G smallest for volume resuscitation, blood and colloids
- grey – 16G
- orange – 14G.

A 45-year-old woman has been diagnosed with metastatic breast cancer and requires repeated administration of intravenous chemotherapy. She has poor peripheral veins.

H   There are a number of long-term central venous cannulation systems available for patients requiring prolonged intravenous drug administration. These are usually tunnelled under the skin for a short distance to reduce the risk of line infection. They should be used with full aseptic precautions. The *Hickman line* is a single-lumen soft cannula which is tunnelled under the skin with the distal end projecting out of the skin. The *portacath system* is a completely subcutaneous system with an injection reservoir buried beneath the skin. The *permacath* is a tunnelled long-term line for renal replacement therapy. A *vascath* is an untunnelled short-term central venous access catheter for renal replacement therapy.

A baby is admitted with severe diarrhoea and needs urgent resuscitation as his consciousness level is deteriorating. The team is unable to find a vein to insert an intravenous cannula.

D   An intraosseous needle should be placed into the tibial medulla approximately 1–3 cm below the tibial tuberosity in the event of failure to gain intravenous access during a paediatric resuscitation. It can be used for the administration of drugs and fluids. The needle should be secured in place and fluids or drugs syringed in with a 20-mL or 50-mL syringe. The main problem is dislodgement of the needle and extravasation of fluid. Longer term complications include development of osteomyelitis.

A patient is in ITU with septic shock. He needs access to deliver noradrenaline (norepinephrine) infusion to increase his blood pressure. He has a large cannula in the dorsum of the hand.

E Central venous access should be established to optimize filling pressures and allow the administration of vasoactive drugs. Noradrenaline should be given through a central line because of the risk of extravasation leading to tissue necrosis.

The anaesthetist would like intravenous access for the induction of anaesthesia in a fit and well adult.

B A 22G or 20G cannula is sufficient for establishing intravenous access in a healthy adult. The smaller cannulae cause less pain. If a large-bore cannula is needed for volume replacement this can be inserted after anaesthesia has been induced. In elderly, unfit or sick patients, large intravenous cannulation should be established before induction in order to allow for treatment of hypotension on induction.

87 Pain relief

ANSWERS: 1B, 2A, 3H, 4I

An 18-year-old man with a diagnosis of osteosarcoma has been admitted to the cardiothoracic unit for removal of a metastasis in his right upper lung lobe. He requires a thoracotomy.

B Epidural analgesia improves morbidity in the high-risk patient and in major surgery such as a thoracotomy as the epidural infusion is usually based on a local anaesthetic in combination with an opioid (fentanyl). The level of epidural analgesia is dependent on the dermatomal level needed to cover the surgical incision.

A 70-year-old day surgery patient needs analgesia prescribing following unilateral varicose vein surgery. The only past medical history of note is occasional complaints of heartburn.

A Postoperative pain peaks initially and consequently eases. The analgesic ladder (WHO) is used as a guide to treat acute postoperative pain. Pain may be assessed using a verbal analogue score (VRS) to guide appropriate therapy: 0 = no pain; 1 = mild pain; 2 = moderate pain; 3 = severe pain; 4 = worst pain. Different operations are estimated to have different pain scores:

- mild to moderate pain (e.g. varicose vein surgery, hysteroscopy)
- moderate to severe pain (e.g. inguinal hernia repair, appendicectomy)
- worst pain (e.g. thoracotomy, nephrectomy, laparotomy).

Balanced analgesia is a principle of pain management; i.e using non-opioid analgesics such as paracetamol and non-steroidal anti-inflammatory drugs (NSAIDs) alongside strong opioids. NSAIDs must be used with caution and may be contraindicated, for example, in patients with renal impairment or gastrointestinal ulceration.

A 65-year-old man with colon cancer requires an anterior resection. He has a significant history of chronic obstructive airways disease treated with high-dose inhaled steroids and aminophylline. His peak expiratory flow rate is 195 mL/s. An ITU bed has been booked for his postoperative recovery.

H   This patient has a high risk for developing respiratory complications and adequate analgesia is vital as abdominal surgery pain will affect the patient's ability to cough up secretions and ventilate appropriately in the postoperative period. The use of epidural anaesthesia is also associated with less opioid use, which is desirable due to the respiratory suppressant effect of large doses of opiates.

A 45-year-old woman is undergoing a left-sided mastectomy for breast cancer. She is very anxious and particularly worried about her postoperative pain as, for previous wide-local excision surgery, she had to wait for her pain-relieving medication.

I   For severe and worst pain, invasive/parenteral analgesia is required and strong opioids can be administered via patient-controlled analgesia (PCA with morphine as the drug of choice). PCA allows patients more control over delivery of analgesia with the ability to deliver bolus injections. There may be a background infusion. There is a limit to the size of the boluses and only a fixed preset amount of opiate can be delivered over a period of time to prevent overdosage.

88 Drugs for anaesthesia

ANSWERS: 1F, 2D, 3E, 4B

A 16-year-old male has been admitted to the A&E department with a diagnosis of acute appendicitis. The surgical team decides to proceed to appendicectomy immediately. After assessing the patient the anaesthetist plans to perform a rapid sequence intubation.

F   Suxamethonium is a short-acting depolarizing muscle relaxant of rapid onset (45 s). It is the drug of choice in this situation, where the airway needs to be secured rapidly to reduce the risk of aspiration.

A 24-year-old woman is scheduled to undergo varicose vein surgery. She is a fit non-smoker and drinks 6 units of alcohol a week. Her last meal was 6 hours ago. The anaesthetist picks a drug for intravenous induction of anaesthesia.

D   Propofol is the most commonly used intravenous induction agent at a dose of 2 mg/kg. It is administered intravenously and consciousness is lost within 30 seconds and waking occurs after 10 minutes following a single dose. As it suppresses airway reflexes it is an excellent choice when a laryngeal mask airway is used to secure the airway. It causes a reduction in blood pressure, systemic vascular resistance and respiratory depression. Most commonly pain on injection is a problem. It can also be used for sedation during intensive care or minor procedures.

Ketamine is an NMDA antagonist and can be used as a induction agent but has unpredictable onset and offset. Its use is restricted by its psychotropic side-effects ('dissociative anaesthesia').

Midazolam is one of the most frequently used benzodiazepines for sedation. Its main actions are for hypnosis, sedation, anxiolysis and anterograde amnesia. The action is linked to GABA receptors. It is short-acting due to its lipophilicity and rapid rate of elimination. However it is not commonly used as an induction agent.

A 6-year-old girl scheduled for a tonsillectomy is severely needle-phobic. It is felt that although an intravenous anaesthetic would be preferable, in this particular situation it would be too traumatic. After discussion with the mother and child, the anaesthetist has offered the choice of a 'gas induction'.

E   'Gas induction' refers to inducing anaesthesia by gases alone. This does not require instant intravenous access. It is used in needle-phobic patients or in a situation where the airway might be of particular concern. Historically it was the first route to induce anaesthesia (Schimmelbusch mask).

Sevoflurane is a modern flurane vapour with advantages of rapid onset and offset, with little irritation to the airway. Cyclopropane has been well tolerated but is now obsolete (it is a flammable anaesthetic agent and its use is discouraged).

A 51-year-old woman is scheduled for a hysterectomy. The surgeons request muscle relaxation. She has been nil by mouth for 10 hours and has no risk of aspirating.

B   Most muscle relaxants are non-depolarizing and competitive antagonists to acetylcholine at the neuromuscular junction. They differ in their onset time, metabolism and side-effects. Tubocurare was much used in the past but is of slow onset and has marked ganglionic adverse effects such as hypotension. Atracurium is more commonly used and has an onset time of 90 seconds. Histamine release may occur with doses of atracurium greater than 0.6 mg/kg. It is broken down spontaneously by Hoffmann's degradation.

89 Oxygen therapy

ANSWERS: 1C, 2G, 3F, 4H

A 20-year-old man was been knocked from his motorbike. He has a clear and patent airway. Examination reveals a possible fractured pelvis and right femur.

C   This patient is likely to be hypovolaemic from loss of blood into his fractures. The priority while he is being resuscitated is to maintain oxygen delivery to the tissues. Tissue oxygenation depends on oxygen content of the blood, delivery and consumption.

Oxygen content of the blood (millilitres of O_2 per 100 mL of blood) is calculated from: $(Hb \times \% Sat \times 1.36) + (PO_2 \times 0.0031)$. In simple terms, this means that tissue oxygenation depends on adequate delivery of oxygen to the haemoglobin and an adequate circulation of oxygenated haemoglobin.

It is difficult to predict inspired oxygen concentration (FiO_2) in spontaneously breathing patients. Simple facemasks (e.g. Hudson) or nasal cannulae will provide 35–55 per cent. Fixed-performance devices can produce a more accurate oxygen delivery. The non-rebreathe mask with reservoir bag is thought to provide the highest FiO_2 without using a sealed facemask. It can produce FiO_2 up to 85 per cent with flow rates of 15 L/min. The reservoir provides a store of oxygen from which the patient inspires during peak inspiratory flow rates. A one-way valve prevents expired gases filling the reservoir bag.

A 65-year-old man with COPD was admitted to the ward with an infective exacerbation of COPD. Pulse oximetry shows 87 per cent oxygen saturation on air. He has a letter from his chest physician which he has been told to keep with him at all times. It describes that the patient relies on a hypoxic ventilatory drive.

G   Patients with chronic pulmonary disease sometimes develop a persistently elevated carbon dioxide level and hypoxia becomes their main stimulation to breathing. Oxygen therapy has to be carefully managed as slight increases in inspired oxygen concentration could cause a respiratory arrest. These patients should carry a medical alert note.

It is vital to avoid hypoxia, so the preferred delivery of oxygen should be via a fixed-performance device at a FiO_2 of 28 per cent. A Venturi mask is a common device that entrains a fixed proportion of oxygen.

If the patient deteriorates requiring increasing FiO_2 above 60 per cent to maintain a PaO_2 above 8 kPa, intubation and ventilation has to be considered.

A 67-year-old man develops shortness of breath, wheeze and is coughing up frothy red sputum. His oxygenation is deteriorating as he is transferred to ITU.

F   Continuous positive airway pressure (CPAP) will supply positive airway pressure throughout all phases of spontaneous ventilation. It is applied via a tight fitting mask. CPAP will increase the functional residual capacity, thereby reducing airway collapse and increasing arterial oxygenation. It is used in weaning from ventilation, chronic airway collapse and pulmonary oedema to improve oxygenation.

A 25-year-old woman is admitted to A&E with an acute exacerbation of her asthma. Examination reveals wheeze throughout both lung fields.

H   Nebulizers are devices to provide a suspension of droplets in a gas for administration of inhaled drugs or humidification. Droplets of 5 nm are deposited in the trachea and smaller ones in the alveoli. Ideal droplet size is 1–5 nm. In asthma, nebulizers are used to enable bronchodilating drugs such as salbutamol (or in severe cases adrenaline (epinephrine)) to reach the bronchi.

90 Preoperative investigation

ANSWERS: 1A, 2C, 3G, 4H

A 75-year-old man with a history of smoking 10–15 cigarettes a day for 35 years is admitted for elective major surgery. He has a productive cough.

A   This investigation is essential in any patient with a significant history of respiratory or cardiac disease or signs on clinical examination scheduled for major surgery. A chest x-ray (CXR) is useful as an indication of structural abnormalities in these conditions but shows less about function. A CXR is indicated as above unless there is a film available within 6–12 months. Other indications include new/change in symptoms, possible metastasis, or recent immigration from an area where tuberculosis is endemic. It also is a preoperative baseline for major surgery and some anaesthetists request a CXR in all elderly patients.

A patient is scheduled for an anterior resection. He has COPD and complains that he has had more chest tightness recently. You wish to assess his lung function in the pre-assessment clinic.

C   Peak flow can be measured with a Wright spirometer as a simple bedside test for obstructive lung disease. This can be indicative of the patient's ability to cough and expectorate secretions. The result is dependent on the patient's weight, but for a 70-kg male less than 200 mL/min indicates significant impairment. This test is also to be repeated after bronchodilators have been administered to assess the reversibility of the disease. Lung function tests are generally used to determine the nature and extent of pulmonary disorders. Measurement of static lung volumes are cumbersome. A spirometer is used to measure forced expiration and derived variables. The ratio of FEV_1/FVC is reduced in obstructive lung disease and normal or high in restrictive lung disease. Flow volume loops will give the anaesthetist an indication of the compliance of the lungs.

A 75-year-old woman attends the pre-assessment clinic prior to total hip replacement. She has had episodes of shortness of breath, chest pain and syncope.

G   Cardiac imaging uses reflection of ultrasound pulses. It is most useful to diagnose and/or quantify valvular heart disease, myocardial and pericardial disease and cardiac function. It can be useful in estimating ejection fraction and cardiac output.

A patient is admitted for vascular surgery to improve the blood flow to his right leg. He is functionally severely compromised. He reports that he has started to get chest pains when he walks for over 30 yards.

H   Electrocardiogram (ECG) is used for investigation of cardiac disease, particularly ischaemic heart disease and arrhythmias. It is an important preoperative investigation in a patient with a history of cardiac disease and it is recommended in the patient over 55 years of age. The ECG is also monitored during anaesthesia (lead II).

91 Support in critical care

ANSWERS: 1I, 2F, 3H, 4B, 5A

A 58-year-old man presents with central chest pain radiating into his back. He has a heart rate 95/min, BP 170/95 mmHg and poor urine output. ECG is normal. He is awaiting a CT scan of his chest.

I   This patient has the classical description of a leaking thoracic aortic aneurysm. Treatment should be aimed at stabilization of his blood pressure while a definitive diagnosis is made. He is hypertensive with a reasonable heart rate. Analgesia should be given to treat his pain and also to lower his blood pressure. If this does not control his blood pressure then a labetalol infusion would be a useful treatment option as it has both α- and β-adrenergic receptor blocking effects. GTN acts as a venodilator and may not control his blood pressure effectively. It will also not slow his heart rate. Once the patient's blood pressure is controlled then cautious fluid challenges may be given to correct the poor urine output.

A 70-year-old diabetic Asian woman presents with intermittent central chest pain. She is on GTN, insulin and a heparin infusion in the cardiac unit. Coronary angiogram shows severe triple-vessel disease. She is awaiting a coronary artery bypass graft but presents with further chest pain in the night. Pulse 70/min, BP 90/50 mmHg, troponin T 0.05.

F   This woman has poor myocardial perfusion secondary to her coronary artery disease. If her myocardial oxygen demands increase she will be unable to increase myocardial oxygen delivery and her myocardium will become more ischaemic and contract poorly. This in turn worsens the situation. She needs her blood pressure supported to maintain coronary perfusion without increasing myocardial oxygen demand.

The intra-aortic counter-pulsation balloon pump is the ideal inotrope in patients with a competent aortic valve. During diastole it inflates to increase coronary perfusion pressure and during systole it deflates reducing the afterload of the heart. All chemical inotropes increase myocardial oxygen demand and are potentially arrhythmogenic.

A 28-year-old male intravenous drug abuser is admitted to ITU with a red, inflamed mass in his groin. He is due to go to theatre to have the mass explored. Heart rate is 115/min, BP 80/30 mmHg, and he is oliguric.

H   Before initiating inotropes, intravascular fluid deficits should be corrected. This young man may well need a vasoconstrictor to maintain his blood pressure in the near future, but using drugs (e.g. noradrenaline) in an inadequately filled circulation can lead to end-organ ischaemia.

A 35-year-old man with septic shock is being treated in ITU. His mean arterial blood pressure has dropped to 65 mmHg despite adequate fluid resuscitation.

B   Noradrenaline (norepinephrine) is a catecholamine that is an immediate precursor of adrenaline (epinephrine). It is a neurotransmitter in the sympathetic nervous system and predominantly stimulates the α-adrenergic response. It is mainly used as an inotropic drug when systemic vascular resistance is low, as in sepsis.

An 8-year-old girl has a cardiopulmonary arrest following a bee sting.

A   Adrenaline is the drug of choice in anaphylaxis. Anaphylaxis is associated with massive vasodilatation causing a significant drop in blood pressure. Adrenaline is a beta-agonist (mainly β1) and alpha-agonist, so it is positively chronotropic and inotropic, and acts to vasoconstrict the circulation. Caution should be taken with the concentration as it is usually available in both 1:1000 and 1:10000 ampoules.

92 Risks and side-effects of general anaesthesia

ANSWERS: 1A, 2E, 3H, 4G, 5C

The risk of sore throat following an anaesthetic.

A   The risk of a sore throat following general anaesthesia depends on the type of airway used: about 1 in 5 with an LMA and 2 in 5 for an endotracheal tube.

The risk of awareness during anaesthesia.

E   Many patients fear awareness during anaesthesia. Up to 1 in 1000
         experience some form of awareness but it may be as rare as 1 in
         42 000. There are different types of awareness. Conscious awareness
         with explicit recall and severe pain occurs in < 1:3000 general
         anaesthetics.

The risk of getting hepatitis B following a blood transfusion.

H   NHS guidelines of the risk of developing a viral infection from a blood
         transfusion is very rare; the risk of getting hepatitis B is about 1 in
         670 000, hepatitis C is about 1 in 82 million and HIV is about 1 in
         5 million

The risk of death during anaesthesia.

G   The risk of death following anaesthesia is rare and it may be difficult
         to ascertain whether anaesthesia was the cause or a contributory factor.
         For young, healthy patients undergoing elective surgery this risk is
         around 1 in 100 000 but this increases 5–10 fold in high-risk patients
         and emergency surgery.

The risk of failed intubation in the obstetric population.

C   There are many definitions of difficult intubation. One includes
         a 'Cormack and Lehane' view of the larynx during laryngoscopy
         where only the epiglottis is seen (i.e. the vocal cords cannot be seen).
         The overall incidence is approximately 5 per cent. However, failed
         intubation (placement of the endotracheal tube fails after multiple
         intubation attempts) is much rarer: in the general surgical group this
         occurs in 1 in 2000 (0.05 per cent); whereas, in obstetric patients, it
         occurs in approximately 1 in 300 patients (0.3 per cent).

93 Anaphylaxis

ANSWERS 1A, 2D, 3H, 4L

         A 20-year-old man is being given intravenous co-amoxiclav
         on the ward and has sudden-onset rash, urticaria, hypotension,
         wheeze, bronchospasm and oedema. What are your first steps in the
         management of this man?

A   Anaphylaxis is a severe, life-threatening, generalized or systemic
         hypersensitivity reaction. It may affect the airway (pharyngeal and
         laryngeal oedema, hoarse voice and stridor), breathing (dyspnoea,
         wheeze and bronchospasm) and circulation (pale, clammy, hypotension,
         tachycardia and cardiac arrest). There may also be gastrointestinal
         symptoms (vomiting, abdominal pain and incontinence) and mucosal/
         skin changes (erythema, urticaria and oedema).

What is the lifetime incidence of anaphylaxis in the UK population?

D   Available UK estimates suggest that approximately 1 in 1333 of the population of England has experienced anaphylaxis at some point in their lives. International data suggests there are between 30 and 950 cases per 100 000 persons per year.

What is the appropriate dose of adrenaline (epinephrine) and its administration route for the treatment of life-threatening anaphylaxis?

H   Adrenaline is given i.m. unless experienced with intravenous adrenaline. For adults, intramuscular doses of 500 mcg (0.5 mL of 1:1000) adrenaline are administered and may be repeated after 5 min if no better. In experienced hands, adrenaline is administered intravenously in increments of 50 mcg (0.5 mL of 1:10 000 solution) intravenously. Several doses may be required if there is severe hypotension or bronchospasm.

What serum indicators are used in the diagnosis of anaphylaxis?

L   The specific test to help confirm a diagnosis of an anaphylactic reaction is measurement of serum tryptase. Tryptase is the major protein component of mast cell secretory granules and is released during anaphylaxis. Blood samples (5–10 mL clotted blood) are taken as soon as possible after resuscitation has started and a second sample is taken 1–2 hours after the start of symptoms. Finally a third sample is taken at 24 hours – this is a measure of baseline tryptase levels as some patients have higher baseline values.

94 Anaesthetic emergencies

ANSWERS: 1D, 2B, 3A, 4J

An obese 40-year-old woman undergoes examination under anaesthetic for an anal fissure. She is induced with propofol and alfentanil. Anaesthesia is maintained with isoflurane. She is lightly anaesthetized in a head-down position with a laryngeal mask airway in place and a clear airway. Ten minutes after the procedure has commenced, she develops marked stridor and reduction in tidal volumes.

D   Laryngospasm can occur from direct stimulation of the vocal cords or as a response to noxious stimulation at a different site. The airway reflexes are increased during the excitatory phase of anaesthesia (i.e. during induction and emergence). Any secretions, blood or instrumentation stimulating the cords may lead to spasm. Indirect laryngospasm can occur during a painful procedure if the depth of anaesthesia or degree of analgesia is inadequate. This patient was induced with two short-acting agents which would have worn off by the time of surgical stimulation and she was lightly anaesthetized with isoflurane. The management of the patient would be to increase oxygen to 100 per cent, maintain CPAP and deepen anaesthesia.

A 40-year-old woman is undergoing emergency surgery for a comminuted tibial fracture. While the surgeon is manipulating the fracture, the anaesthetist notices a sudden loss of end tidal carbon dioxide trace.

B   Any loss of the end tidal carbon dioxide trace should be taken seriously. Usually it is due to equipment issues such as a blocked sampling line or disconnection. However, if cardiac output is significantly reduced then CO_2 delivery to the lungs falls and a drop in the end tidal CO_2 level will be noted. In the event of a massive pulmonary embolism the first sign may be loss of the end tidal CO_2.

A 24-year-old woman is undergoing a diagnostic laparoscopy. She has never had a general anaesthetic before. Following intravenous induction, anaesthesia is maintained with isoflurane. The patient develops a sudden tachycardia. A rapid increase in the end tidal carbon dioxide trace is noted.

A   Malignant hyperthermia is an autosomal dominant condition resulting in a defective ryanodine receptor. This is a calcium efflux channel in the sarcoplasmic reticulum. On exposure to triggering agents such as volatile anaesthetic agents and suxamethonium there is muscle rigidity and increased metabolism. The first signs include an unexplained increase in heart rate and rising end tidal CO_2.

A 70-year-old woman has difficulty breathing after extubation following a general anaesthetic for an umbilical hernia repair. She had been intubated and ventilated following 100 mg of propofol, 10 mg of vecuronium and 100 mcg of fentanyl. Anaesthesia was maintained with isoflurane and a further 4 mg of vecuronium was administered 15 minutes before extubation.

J   Incomplete reversal of muscle relaxants can present in a variety of ways. The patient may be seen to be making respiratory effort but their tidal volumes may be inadequate to clear carbon dioxide. As a result CO_2 levels rise leading to a reduction in consciousness and a worsening respiratory acidosis. This woman received a large dose of vecuronium and reversal was attempted within 35 minutes of the beginning of the procedure.

Incomplete reversal may sometimes present with an agitated patient with reduced power making 'fish out of water' type movements.

SECTION 8: PLASTIC SURGERY

QUESTIONS

95 Assessment of burns

A	9 per cent	G	10 per cent
B	45 per cent	H	5 per cent
C	80 per cent	I	15 per cent
D	36 per cent	J	1 per cent
E	60 per cent	K	20 per cent
F	18 per cent	L	54 per cent

For each clinical scenario below choose the approximate percentage total burn surface area. Each option may be used only once.

1   A 24-year-old man is rescued from a house fire and has suffered extensive partial-thickness burns to the whole of his back and the posterior aspect of both legs.

2   A 16-year-old male suffers partial-thickness burns to the palm of his right hand.

3   An 8-year-old girl pulls a kettle of boiling water over herself, suffering full-thickness burns to her anterior trunk.

4   A 64-year-old engineer is involved in a major gas explosion, suffering full-thickness burns over the head and neck and partial-thickness burns to chest, abdomen and arms.

Answers: see page 231

96 Complications of burns

A   hypovolaemia
B   contractures
C   deep vein thrombosis
D   rhabdomyolysis
E   Curling's ulcer
F   type II respiratory failure
G   type I respiratory failure

H   acute myocardial infarction
I   disseminated intravascular coag-
    ulation
J   hypothermia
K   toxic shock syndrome
L   compartment syndrome

For each clinical scenario below choose the most likely complication. Each option may be used only once.

1   A 45-year-old woman is brought to A&E after being rescued from a house fire. On examination she has suffered partial-thickness burns to both arms and full-thickness burns to her chest and the soles of her feet. She is distressed and coughs up soot as she asks to see her family. Respiratory rate is 33/min with poor chest expansion. Pulse oximetry is 94 per cent (15 L/min O_2 through non-rebreathe mask). Auscultation of the chest reveals poor air entry bilaterally with no added sounds.

2   A 35-year-old man is being monitored on the burns unit after suffering full-thickness burns to his hands secondary to high-voltage electrocution. Urinalysis reveals microscopic haematuria. Blood tests reveal a mild hyperkalaemia and a creatinine kinase (CK) of 3000 U/L.

3   A 2-year-old child is brought to A&E acutely unwell by her mother 48 hours after suffering a scald to the right forearm. On examination there is a Flama-zine dressing over the burn site. The patient is pyrexial and tachycardic with a low blood pressure.

4   A 47-year-old man with a full-thickness circumferential burn to the left arm complains of persistent pain refractory to morphine analgesia. On examination radial and brachial pulses are palpable and the arm is too painful to examine.

Answers: see page 232

97 Skin cover

A   split-thickness skin graft   E   pedicled myocutaneous flap
B   full-thickness skin graft   F   sterile skin closure strips
C   healing by secondary intention   G   primary closure with sutures
D   local flap   H   free flap

For each clinical scenario below choose the most appropriate means of reconstruction. Each option may be used only once.

1   A 74-year-old woman presents to A&E with a small proximally based preti-bial laceration with no soft tissue loss. She is known to have ischaemic heart disease, COPD and diabetes.

2   A 44-year-old woman would like breast reconstruction surgery following a right-sided mastectomy and postoperative radiotherapy. She is known to be a non-insulin-dependent diabetic and previously smoked 20 cigarettes a day.

3   A 25-year-old patient has suffered a full-thickness burn over the posterior aspect of her trunk.

4   A 43-year-old woman presents with a biopsy-proven 3 cm × 3 cm squamous cell carcinoma over the right side of her forehead. Tumour excision included the periosteum of the skull. The patient is particularly concerned about the cosmetic outcome.

Answers: see page 233

ANSWERS

95 Assessment of burns

ANSWERS: 1D, 2J, 3F, 4B

The Wallace *rule of nines* is a simple and rough guide to assessing the extent of burn injuries. The body is divided into 10 anatomical regions that are multiples of 9 per cent (see Figure 95.1). The perineum is estimated as 1 per cent, as is the palmar surface of the hand, which is an alternative way of assessing percentage body area involved. The most accurate method of assessing total body surface area (TBSA) involved is the Lund and Browder chart which is used in burns units. It is important to remember that the rule of nines needs to be modified when applied to a child as the head represents a larger surface area and the legs represent a smaller surface area compared to an adult.

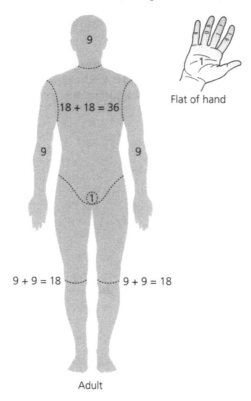

Fig. 95.1 Reproduced with permission from Patel, K. 2012: *Complete Revision Notes for Medical and Surgical Finals,* Second edition. London: Hodder Arnold.

Although each case should be considered individually, it is suggested that burns > 10 per cent of TBSA in adults and > 5 per cent of TBSA in children should be referred to a burns centre. The other criteria for referral are: burns involving face, hands, feet, genitalia, perineum, full-thickness burns > 5 per cent, electrical and chemical burns, burns with associated inhalation injury and circumferential burns.

The TBSA affected is used to guide intravenous fluid resuscitation of the burns patient. Resuscitation is started if the burn involves > 15 per cent of TBSA in adults and > 10 per cent of TBSA in children. There are a number of formulae that can be used to estimate the fluid requirement.

- Current *ATLS guidelines* suggest that 2–4 mL × bodyweight (kg) × per cent TBSA should be administered in the first 24 hours. For example, a 70 kg man with 20 per cent TBSA burns will require 2800–5600 mL in the first 24 hours. Half of this should be provided in the first 8 hours after the injury and the remainder given in the final 16 hours.
- The *Muir and Barclay formula* (preferred by UK burns units and using human albumin solution) describes a formula for fluid resuscitation for the first 36 hours after burn injury: replacement volume (mL) = 0.5 × bodyweight (kg) × per cent TBSA. This replacement volume should be given 4-hourly for the first 12 hours, 6-hourly for the next 12 hours, and 12-hourly for the final 12 hours.

It is important to recognize that all formulae are merely estimates and the patient's response to fluid (e.g. urine output) needs to be assessed continuously to guide resuscitation.

96 Complications of burns

ANSWERS: 1F, 2D, 3K, 4L

A 45-year-old woman is brought to A&E after being rescued from a house fire. On examination she has suffered partial-thickness burns to both arms and full-thickness burns to her chest and the soles of her feet. She is distressed and coughs up soot as she asks to see her family. Respiratory rate is 33/min with poor chest expansion. Pulse oximetry is 94 per cent (15 L/min O_2 through non-rebreathe mask). Auscultation of the chest reveals poor air entry bilaterally with no added sounds.

F   There can be significant airway and breathing problems in patients presenting with burns. Patients with inhalation burn injury may present initially with subtle symptoms and signs and so there should be a low threshold for intervention. The concern is development of significant upper airway oedema/obstruction that necessitates difficult provision of an emergency airway. Soot around the nose/mouth and burns/swelling around the lips is suggestive of airway burn. Airway oedema is progressive in the first 24 hours and so prophylactic intubation must be considered.

In this particular patient there are full-thickness burns to the chest wall with accompanying reduced chest expansion and air entry. The burn injury has impaired the compliance of the chest wall causing respiratory embarrassment which results in type II respiratory failure (i.e. ventilatory failure). An arterial blood gas may well show hypercapnia due to reduced ability to expire CO_2 that is consequently retained. Urgent escharotomy is required to increase chest wall compliance.

Type I respiratory failure may also develop from carbon monoxide poisoning. It is important to obtain an early baseline carboxyhaemoglobin reading and to persist with maximal oxygen therapy. Arterial PO_2 measurements do not reliably predict carbon monoxide poisoning. Patients with serious burns are also at risk of developing type I respiratory failure from other mechanisms (e.g. pulmonary oedema and acute lung injury).

A 35-year-old man is being monitored on the burns unit after suffering full-thickness burns to his hands secondary to high-voltage electrocution. Urinalysis reveals microscopic haematuria. Blood tests reveal a mild hyperkalaemia and a creatinine kinase (CK) of 3000 U/L.

D   Risk of development of rhabdomyolysis should always be considered in a patient with electrocution injury. This is more likely with high-voltage (> 1000 V) than domestic voltage injuries.

Rhabdomyolysis involves the breakdown of muscle fibres with the consequent release of potentially toxic intracellular contents into plasma. The CK is characteristically raised several times above the reference range. There may be hyperkalaemia due to release from muscle. Urinalysis that is positive for blood but negative for red blood cells implies myoglobinuria and is suggestive of rhabdomyolysis. The urine has a characteristically dark appearance. Acute renal failure may develop secondary to hypovolaemia and acute tubular necrosis which is caused by toxic free radical products from myoglobin (these are formed under acidic conditions). The myoglobin casts themselves may also cause tubular obstruction.

Prompt treatment with intravenous fluid resuscitation and reversal of the acidosis is crucial in treating impending renal failure.

A 2-year-old child is brought to A&E acutely unwell by her mother 48 hours after suffering a scald to the right forearm. On examination there is a Flamazine dressing over the burn site. The patient is pyrexial and tachycardic with a low blood pressure.

K   Toxic shock syndrome (TSS) is a systemic inflammatory response syndrome that is usually caused by dissemination of a staphylococcal exotoxin. Burns and scalds damage the normal skin defences, increasing the susceptibility to infection. Antibodies directed at TSS toxin usually develop by early childhood, protecting the patient from the full cytokine cascade response. However, these antibodies are often not developed in younger children, increasing the risk of TSS (particularly in children younger than 3 years). Therefore there should be a low threshold for admission and treatment of children with minor burns who present acutely unwell in the first few days following a burn injury.

A 47-year-old man with a full-thickness circumferential burn to the left arm complains of persistent pain refractory to morphine analgesia. On examination radial and brachial pulses are palpable and the arm is too painful to examine.

L   There is a particularly high risk of developing compartment syndrome following full-thickness circumferential burns to a limb as the burned skin acts like a tourniquet. The classical finding is significantly increasing analgesia requirements that are disproportionate to the injury. There is pain elicited on passive stretching of the affected compartment muscles and the patient often complains of paraesthesia. The pulses may be present until very high intracompartmental pressures develop, so pulselessness should not be relied on as a clinical sign. Intracompartmental pressures may be measured, but the diagnosis is principally clinical. Urgent fasciotomy/escharotomy is indicated.

97 Skin cover

ANSWERS: 1F, 2H, 3A, 4D

A 74-year-old woman presents to A&E with a small proximally based pretibial laceration with no soft tissue loss. She is known to have ischaemic heart disease, COPD and diabetes.

F   The skin over the tibia is susceptible to injury particularly in the elderly as the skin is thin and inelastic with little subcutaneous soft tissue padding. Management can be either conservative or surgical. Conservative closure with sterile adhesive strips is preferred to suturing as they put the healing tissue under less tension and sutures often tend to pull through. This is probably the best course of action in the first instance in this scenario as the patient poses a significant anaesthetic risk. Should the flap necrose then surgical management involves debridement of devitalized tissue and split skin grafting.

A 44-year-old woman would like breast reconstruction surgery following a right-sided mastectomy and postoperative radiotherapy. She is known to be a non-insulin-dependent diabetic and previously smoked 20 cigarettes a day.

H   There a number of options available for reconstruction of any area and there is a huge range for the reconstruction of breasts. These can be carried out at the time of mastectomy (i.e. immediate) or at a later date (i.e. delayed). The timing of surgery depends on the patient's and surgeon's preference.

Either a pedicled flap or a free flap may be used to reconstruct tissue defects. A *pedicled flap* involves mobilizing tissue (muscle with skin and fat) on its blood supply and siting into the new position without interrupting the blood supply. An example of this with regard to breast reconstruction is a latissimus dorsi pedicled flap. A *free flap* involves detaching the tissue (interrupting the blood supply), reimplanting at the recipient site and performing a vascular anastomosis to the local blood supply. An example of this with regard to breast reconstruction is the TRAM (transverse rectus abdominis myocutaneous) free flap.

The type of reconstruction involves close discussion between surgeon and patient. A free TRAM flap will give a superior cosmetic result and tends to have the better blood supply, and in a patient with microvascular insufficiency (smoker, diabetic) this would be the preferred option. Also the latissimus dorsi reconstruction often requires an implant to achieve sufficient volume, which is at risk of becoming infected given the patient's diabetes.

A 25-year-old patient has suffered a full-thickness burn over the posterior aspect of her trunk.

A   A graft is a unit of tissue(s) that is transplanted to a new site independent of blood supply. A *split-thickness graft* (STG) consists of the epidermis with a varying amount of dermis, as opposed to a *full-thickness graft* (FTG) which contains the entire thickness of dermis.

An STG is useful for covering large areas due to larger donor areas. An STG is harvested usually from the patient's thigh using a dermatome. The donor site then heals by re-epithelialization. The disadvantage of STG is that there is increased contraction and poor cosmesis in comparison to an FTG. The donor site of STG can also be slow to heal.

An FTG is useful for smaller areas where cosmesis is important and contraction would be problematic (e.g. volar aspect of digits). They are less likely to 'take' and are limited in size as the secondary defect needs to be closed directly.

In the scenario given, a large area needs coverage and so an STG is the more practical option.

A 43-year-old woman presents with a biopsy-proven 3 cm × 3 cm squamous cell carcinoma over the right side of her forehead. Tumour excision included the periosteum of the skull. The patient is particularly concerned about the cosmetic outcome.

D   In this case, primary closure of the defect will not be possible. An FTG will provide a reasonable cosmetic result but will not 'take' on bone (grafts require a vascularized bed to 'take', and the periosteum has been resected). The only reconstructive option, which would also provide the best cosmetic outcome, would be a local flap.

There are a number of possible designs for local skin flaps, which depend on the site and size of the defect. In this case, bilateral advancement flaps may be used.

SECTION 9: RADIOLOGY

QUESTIONS

98 Imaging of the acute abdomen

A   plain abdominal radiograph
B   contrast enhanced abdomen and pelvic CT scan – portal venous phase
C   unenhanced CT KUB (Kidneys, ureters and bladder) scan
D   contrast enhanced abdomen and pelvic CT scan – arterial phase
E   ultrasound of the abdomen
F   erect chest radiograph
G   transvaginal ultrasound
H   contrast enhanced abdomen and pelvic CT scan – triple phase (unenhanced followed by arterial and portal venous phase enhancement scans)
I   magnetic resonance cholangio-pancreatography (MRCP)
J   virtual colonoscopy

Select the most appropriate form of imaging for each of the following scenarios.

1   A 35-year-old male presents to the emergency department with acute-onset loin pain. On dipstick he is positive for blood.

2   A 90-year-old male is brought into the emergency department. He is pale, sweating and has a low blood pressure with narrow pulse pressure. A pulsatile, expansile mass can be felt in his abdomen.

3   A 20-year-old woman attends the emergency department with acute lower abdominal pain. A urine pregnancy test performed in the emergency department is positive.

4   An obese 40-year-old woman attends the emergency department with colicky upper abdominal pain. She has had previous episodes after eating.

5   An elderly patient with Alzheimer's disease is brought into the emergency department by his carers. They report that he has not opened his bowels for 4 days and his abdomen has become increasingly distended.

ANSWERS: see page 241

99 Imaging of the chest

A   opacification in the right lower zone with loss of clarity of the right heart border

B   loss of clarity of the left hemi-diaphragm with increased retro-cardiac density

C   a peripheral wedge-shaped area with decreased vascular markings

D   a veil-like opacification over the left hemi-thorax

E   a lumpy enlargement of the hila

F   a globular-shaped appearance to the heart

G   a spiculated mass in the right upper zone

H   increased lucency (consist-ent with air) beneath the right hemidiaphragm

I   a 'boot' shape contour to the heart

J   opacification with loss of clarity of the right hemidiaphragm with a normal appearance to the right heart border

Select the most likely radiological findings for the clinical scenarios below.

1   A 50-year-old male with productive cough, fever and crackles over the left chest posteriorly.

2   An Afro-Caribbean woman with tender red nodules on her shins.

3   A heavy smoker with weight loss of 15 kg in three months and worsening shortness of breath.

4   A 30-year-old woman recently returned to the UK from Japan by aeroplane. She has haemoptysis and a swollen left lower leg.

5   A 50-year-old male with acute abdominal pain; he has guarding and rigidity on palpation.

ANSWERS: see page 242

100 Emergency radiology

A   non-accidental injury
B   large bowel obstruction
C   sigmoid volvulus
D   small bowel obstruction
E   traumatic diaphragmatic
     herniation

F   perforated bowel
G   pathological fracture
H   multiple myeloma
I   subdural haemorrhage
J   extradural haemorrhage
K   subarachnoid haemorrhage

Select the likely diagnosis from the options above for the following clinical scenarios.

1   You are seeing a 1-year-old in the emergency department. You notice fractures of the posterior ribs on the chest radiograph.

2   You are the surgical doctor on call. You see a patient in the emergency department with multiple dilated loops of bowel in the centre of the radiograph.

3   You are the orthopaedic doctor on call. You are asked to see a 90-year-old woman with a fractured neck of femur. You notice a solitary lucent lesion through which the fracture passes.

4   You are the surgical foundation year 1 doctor. You are asked to see a man with severe abdominal pain. You notice that the bowel wall is very clear and easily seen on his abdominal radiograph.

5   You are working in the emergency department. You are reviewing the CT scan of a young man who attended hospital after being hit across the head with a bat. You notice a unilateral lentiform area of high density between the skull and the brain.

ANSWERS: see page 243

101 Radiological investigations

A	CT pulmonary angiogram (CTPA)	G	plain radiograph
B	high-resolution CT (HRCT)	H	CT with contrast in the arterial
C	ultrasound with Doppler imaging		phase
D	MRI of the cervical spine	I	positron emission tomography
E	MRI of the lumbar spine		(PET) scan
F	MRI of the head and spine with	J	ultrasound
	contrast		

For each of the following clinical scenarios choose the most appropriate radiological investigation.

1   A pregnant woman presents with an acutely swollen and red left calf.

2   A 35-year-old woman presents with a mass in the midline of her neck that does not move with tongue protrusion.

3   A 25-year-old woman who has had several years of intermittent neurological symptoms including loss of vision.

4   A 60-year-old man presents with a shooting pain from his back down the back of leg and into the foot.

5   A 16-year-old was playing football when he was tackled badly. He has bruising over the lateral aspect of his foot.

ANSWERS: see page 244

ANSWERS

98 Imaging of the acute abdomen

ANSWERS: 1C, 2D, 3G, 4E, 5A

A 35-year-old male presents to the emergency department with acute-onset loin pain. On dipstick he is positive for blood.

C   This is a classic presentation for renal colic. An unenhanced CT scan will allow the urinary stone to be identified within the renal tract and determine if there is hydroureter or hydronephrosis. Since the stone is high density it may be difficult to see the stone if contrast has been given as contrast is also high density.

A 90-year-old male is brought into the emergency department. He is pale, sweating and has a low blood pressure with narrow pulse pressure. A pulsatile, expansile mass can be felt in his abdomen.

D   This man has all the classical features of a ruptured abdominal aortic aneurysm. An arterial phase CT scan (where the contrast is in the arteries) will allow you to determine the exact size, shape and location of the aneurysm as well as the site of the leak. The scan is performed 30 seconds after the contrast is injected into the vein. This will aid the surgeons in surgical planning and also determine if the patient is feasible for an endovascular repair of the aneurysm.

A 20-year-old woman attends the emergency department with acute lower abdominal pain. A urine pregnancy test performed in the emergency department is positive.

G   This young woman has an ectopic pregnancy. Transvaginal ultrasound is the modality of choice. The absence of an intrauterine pregnancy allows the presumptive diagnosis of ectopic pregnancy to be made in the presence of a raised beta-HCG.

An obese 40-year-old woman attends the emergency department with colicky upper abdominal pain. She has had previous episodes after eating.

E   This woman has classical symptom of biliary colic. An ultrasound of the abdomen can demonstrate gallstones and if there is biliary dilatation. The stones are seen as echogenic masses with a shadow behind them. The gallbladder is normally easily identified along with the intra-hepatic biliary tree. The common bile duct can also be seen at the porta hepatis; however, it can be difficult to see the entire common bile duct. If a stone is causing obstruction at any point, the bile ducts behind the stone are dilated. You may also see gallbladder wall thickening and fluid around the gallbladder.

An elderly patient with Alzheimer's disease is brought into the emergency department by his carers. They report that he has not opened his bowels for 4 days and his abdomen has become increasingly distended.

A This patient is likely to have a sigmoid volvulus. A plain radiograph will show the dilated loop of bowel extending up towards the diaphragm. The classic description of a sigmoid volvulus is of a 'bean' that arises from the pelvis. Predisposing conditions include megacolon, chronic constipation and psychiatric conditions.

99 Imaging of the chest

ANSWERS: 1B, 2E, 3G, 4C, 5H

A 50-year-old male with productive cough, fever and crackles over the left chest posteriorly.

B The description is of left lower lobe pneumonia. Consolidation in the left lower lobe will cause loss of clarity of the left hemidiaphragm. There is increased density behind the heart because of the consolidation. Air bronchograms will also be seen behind the heart.

An Afro-Caribbean woman with tender red nodules on her shins.

E This woman has a likely diagnosis of sarcoidosis. A differential for bilateral hilar enlargement is sarcoidosis. Tuberculosis and lymphoma can also appear as bilateral hilar enlargement. The hila can also be enlarged by vascular causes such as pulmonary hypertension; however, the enlargement tends to be smooth and not lumpy.

A heavy smoker with worsening shortness of breath and weight loss of 15 kg in the last three months.

G This man has a likely diagnosis of lung malignancy and a spiculated mass should always be treated as cancer until proven otherwise. He will need further imaging with CT to aid diagnosis and help with staging of the disease.

A 30-year-old woman recently returned to the UK from Japan by aeroplane. She has haemoptysis and a swollen left lower leg.

C This woman has a pulmonary embolus. Occasionally a wedge-shaped area of increased lucency can be seen which is caused by decreased vascular markings in the area. This is known as Westermark's sign.

A 50-year-old male with acute abdominal pain; he has guarding and rigidity on palpation.

H This man has a perforated viscus. Air may be seen under the diaphragm on an erect chest radiograph. In order to maximize the chance of seeing air under the diaphragm the patient must be upright for at least 15 minutes before the radiograph is taken. Air under the diaphragm is seen in only 60% of perforations.

100 Emergency radiology

ANSWERS: 1A, 2D, 3G, 4F, 5J

You are seeing a 1-year-old in the emergency department. You notice fractures of the posterior ribs on the chest radiograph.

A Posterior rib fractures in a child strongly suggest non-accidental injury. If the rib fractures are of different ages then this is highly suggestive and measures to protect the child must be instigated. Other suspicious fractures including metaphyseal corner fractures, sternal fractures, and skull fractures.

You are the surgical doctor on call. You see a patient in the emergency department with multiple dilated loops of bowel in the centre of the radiograph.

D Dilated loops of bowel in the centre of the abdominal radiograph suggest small bowel obstruction. The most common causes of small bowel obstruction include hernia and adhesions.

You are the orthopaedic doctor on call. You are asked to see a 90-year-old woman with a fractured neck of femur. You notice a solitary lucent lesion through which the fracture passes.

G This is a description of a pathological fracture. In this case a primary malignancy such as breast cancer must be sought. Multiple myeloma tends to cause smaller lucent lesions and these cause endosteal scalloping.

You are the surgical foundation year 1 doctor. You are asked to see a man with severe abdominal pain. You notice that the bowel wall is very clear and easily seen on his abdominal radiograph.

F This describes Rigler's sign. Air on both sides of the bowel makes the bowel wall very easy to see and is caused by free intraperitoneal air.

You are working in the emergency department. You are reviewing the CT scan of a young man who attended hospital after being hit across the head with a bat. You notice a unilateral lentiform area of high density between the skull and the brain.

J A unilateral lens-shaped area of high density is the description of an acute extradural haematoma, which is a neurosurgical emergency. It may be caused by rupture of the middle meningeal artery. When interpreting CT imaging it is worth noting that an extradural haematoma will not cross sutures whereas a subdural haemorrhage will cross the cranial sutures.

101 Radiological investigations

ANSWERS: 1C, 2J, 3F, 4E, 5G

A pregnant woman presents with an acutely swollen and red left calf.

C   This woman has a likely diagnosis of deep vein thrombosis. An ultrasound of the lower limb vessels is the first line investigation. The DVT will show up as an echogenic lesion within the deep venous system of the leg and the vein at this point will not be compressible. Radiation should be avoided at all costs during pregnancy especially during the first trimester.

A 35-year-old woman presents with a mass in the midline of her neck that does not move with tongue protrusion.

J   The thyroid gland is a superficial structure and is perfectly amenable to investigation with ultrasound. The ultrasound will determine the size and echotexture of any nodules and also if they are solid or cystic. Certain features on ultrasound are also suspicious for underlying malignancy, e.g. microcalcification. In addition vascularity of the gland can also be assessed.

A 25-year-old woman who has had several years of intermittent neurological symptoms including loss of vision.

F   This woman may be suffering from multiple sclerosis (MS) and needs imaging of her brain and spinal cord. The lesions in MS show up as high-intensity foci on T2 weighted scans and are typically oval-shaped and located adjacent to the ventricles with the orientation of the lesions perpendicular to that of the ventricles.

A 60-year-old man presents with a shooting pain from his back down the back of leg and into the foot.

E   This man is describing a radicular type of pain and this may be caused by a disc prolapse. The imaging modality of choice for looking at the nerves, spinal cord and intervertebral discs is an MRI. The herniated disc is more easily identifiable on T2 weighted scans. If the patient cannot undergo an MRI an alternative imaging technique is a CT myelogram. This involves injecting contrast into the CSF space followed by CT imaging. This will identify the herniated disc compressing the nerve.

A 16-year-old was playing football when he was tackled badly. He has bruising over the lateral aspect of his foot.

G   This young man is likely to have a fracture of the base of his 5th metatarsal and requires plain radiographs for diagnosis. It is unlikely that the fracture will not be seen on plain radiographs and more complicated imaging such as MRI or CT is not warranted in the first instance.

SECTION 10: EMQ REVISION BOXES

The following boxes are directed towards revision for extended matching questions. They concentrate on particular collections of symptoms/signs or phrases to look out for in questions. Answering EMQs is considerably aided by *pattern recognition*, and we hope reading through these boxes encourages you to think along those lines in addition to providing information.

1   Abdominal pain
2   Weight loss
3   Hepatobiliary surgery
4   Chronic liver disease
5   Paediatric surgery
6   Surgical radiology
7   Inflammatory bowel disease
8   Skin lesions
9   Thyroid malignancy
10 Thyroid disease
11 Urology investigations
12 Renal calculi
13 Lump in the groin
14 Dizziness/vertigo

REVISION BOXES

1 Abdominal pain

Box 1 lists the classical abdominal pain descriptions that come up in EMQs.

Box 1 Abdominal pain descriptions

Description	Problem
Colicky loin pain radiating to groin	Ureteric colic
Constant right upper quadrant pain ± jaundice	Biliary colic
Severe epigastric pain radiating to back: Associated with vomiting History of gallstones/↑↑ alcohol	Acute pancreatitis
Periumbilical pain radiating to right iliac fossa	Acute appendicitis
Central abdominal pain, expansile pulsatile mass	Abdominal aortic aneurysm
Iliac fossa pain, positive pregnancy test	Ectopic pregnancy
Severe abdominal pain with rigid abdomen	Perforated viscus

2 Weight loss

As shown in Box 2, weight loss is a classical soft sign towards malignancy in an EMQ.

Box 2 Some associations between weight loss and malignancy

Symptoms	Malignancy
Weight loss, anaemia, dysphagia	Oesophageal carcinoma
Weight loss, painless obstructive jaundice	Pancreatic head carcinoma
Weight loss, haemoptysis, smoker	Bronchial carcinoma
Weight loss, painless haematuria	Bladder carcinoma
Weight loss, change in bowel habit, rectal bleeding	Sigmoid/rectal carcinoma
Flushing, abdominal pain, diarrhoea, heart failure	Carcinoid syndrome

3 Hepatobiliary surgery

The two conditions in Box 3 are frequently confused with each other and commonly crop up in EMQs.

Box 3 Primary biliary cirrhosis and primary sclerosing cholangitis

Presentation	Condition
Middle-aged woman presents with:	Primary biliary cirrhosis
Pruritus, jaundice, pigmentation	
Antimitochondrial antibody positive	
Associated with:	
Rheumatoid arthritis	
Sjögren's syndrome	
Thyroid disease	
Keratoconjunctivitis sicca	
Renal tubular acidosis	
Membranous glomerulonephritis	
Usually middle-aged male:	Primary sclerosing cholangitis
Pruritus, jaundice, abdominal pain	
↑ ALP, antimitochondrial antibody negative	
Associated with inflammatory bowel disease (esp. UC)	

4 Chronic liver disease

Box 4 gives some examples of signs of liver disease particularly relevant to EMQs.

Box 4 Signs of liver disease

Clubbing	
Flapping tremor	
Dupuytren's contracture	
Palmar erythema*	
Gynaecomastia	
Spider naevi*	
*denotes signs that also occur in acute liver disease	
Chronic liver disease associated with:	
Early-onset emphysema	α-1 antitrypsin deficiency
Pigmentation, diabetes	Haemochromatosis
Dysarthria, dyskinesia, dementia, Kayser–Fleischer ring	Wilson's disease

5 Paediatric surgery

Look out for the features in Box 5 in EMQS concerning paediatric surgical presentations.

Box 5 Paediatric signs

Condition	Feature
Pyloric stenosis	Projectile vomiting
	Right upper quadrant mass
Intussusception	Redcurrant jelly stools
Hirschsprung's disease	Failure to pass meconium, distended abdomen
	Absence of air in rectum
Duodenal atresia	Bilious vomiting
	'Double bubble' on x-ray

6 Surgical radiology

Box 6 shows phrases to look out for describing x-ray features in EMQs.

Box 6 X-ray features

X-ray feature	Condition
Free air under diaphragm	Perforated viscus (e.g. diverticulum/duodenal ulcer)
Sentinel loop	Acute pancreatitis
Inverted U loop	Sigmoid volvulus
Loss of haustral pattern	Ulcerative colitis
Cobblestoning	Crohn's disease
Apple-core lesion	Carcinoma of colon

7 Inflammatory bowel disease

Crohn's disease and ulcerative colitis are the two major forms of inflammatory bowel disease. There is significant overlap in the clinical features of these diseases. Box 7 summarizes typical presentations and highlights differing features that are likely to be mentioned in EMQs.

Box 7 Crohn's disease and ulcerative colitis

Can affect anywhere between mouth and anus Skip lesions Weight loss, diarrhoea, abdominal pain Strictures, anal fistulae Barium enema: 'Cobblestoning', 'rose-thorn' ulcers Granulomas	Crohn's disease

Only affects colon
 	
Continuous disease
 	
Diarrhoea with blood and mucus
 	
Fever, tachycardia, toxic megacolon in severe acute UC
 	
Barium enema:
  Loss of haustra
 	
Sigmoidoscopy:
  Oedematous, friable mucosa
 	
No granulomas
	Ulcerative colitis

8 Skin lesions

Look out for particular phrases in questions describing skin lesions. The descriptive features in Box 8 direct you to the likely diagnosis.

Box 8 Characteristic skin lesions

Skin lesion	EMQ feature
Sebaceous cyst	Punctum
Squamous cell carcinoma	Everted edge, lymphadenopathy
Basal cell carcinoma	Rolled, pearly edge
Keratoacanthoma	Central necrotic core, horn projection, spontaneous resolution
Ganglion	Firm swelling moves with tendon (often dorsum of the wrist)
Neurofibroma	Causes tingling, may be multiple
Lipoma	Lobulated, compressible mass
Keloid	Lesion extending beyond scar
Melanoma	Itchy, bleeding, changing shape/colour

9 Thyroid malignancy

Box 9 lists features to look out for in questions concerning thyroid malignancy.

Box 9 Features of thyroid cancer

Thyroid cancer	Features
Follicular carcinoma	Usually woman and solitary lesion
	Haematogenous spread (e.g. bone)
Papillary carcinoma	Often multifocal, early lymph node spread
	Orphan Annie nuclei
	Psammoma bodies
Anaplastic carcinoma	Usually elderly
	Aggressive, so may be rapidly growing mass, airway compression
Medullary carcinoma	May mention associated features of MEN syndrome (e.g. phaeochromocytoma)
Lymphoma	May mention general features: hepatomegaly, splenomegaly, night sweats

10 Thyroid disease

Box 10 lists features to look out for in questions concerning thyroid dysfunction.

Box 10 Thyroid dysfunction

Thyroid condition	EMQ features
Hashimoto's thyroiditis	Hypothyroid symptoms with goitre (e.g. weight gain, bradycardia, constipation)
	Lymphocytic, plasma cell infiltrate, follicles
	Parenchymal atrophy
Graves' disease	Goitre, hyperthyroid, eye signs (e.g. exophthalmos, lid lag)
	Pretibial myxoedema
Endemic goitre	Iodine deficiency, longstanding increased TSH
	Rare in UK
De Quervain's thyroiditis	Tender thyroid, post-viral illness

11 Urology investigations

Box 11 lists common investigations that come up in EMQs.

Box 11 Urology investigations

Investigation	Uses
Ultrasound scan	Evaluation of hydronephrosis, hydroureter and urinary tract stones
Fluoroscopy and video uro-dynamics	Determines bladder, intra–abdominal and urethral pressures
Cystourethroscopy	Visual evaluation in cases of haematuria, persistent post-operative incontinence, and suspected cases of malignan-cy, fistula or diverticulum
Intravenous pyelography	Differentiates between uretero-vesical fistula, vesicovaginal fistula and ureterocoele
Positive-pressure urethrogram	Diagnosing urethral diverticulum
MRI	Visualizing pelvic floor defects

12 Renal calculi

Box 12 lists the incidences and associations of renal calculi.

Box 12 Renal calculi

Calculus	Incidence	Associations
Calcium oxalate	75 per cent	Alkaline urine Disordered calcium metabolism (e.g. hyper-parathyroidism) Increased oxalate absorption (e.g. Crohn's disease)
Triple phosphate	15 per cent	Alkaline urine Urea splitting organisms (e.g. *Proteus*)
Urate	5 per cent	Acidic urine, gout
Cysteine	2 per cent	Acidic urine, cysteine metabolism disorder

13 Lump in the groin

In EMQ presentations of a scrotal/groin swelling, look out for the key features of whether the swelling is distinctively testicular and whether you can palpate above the swelling (see Box 13).

Box 13 Clinical testing of a lump in the groin

When assessing a scrotal swelling:	Can you palpate above the swelling?	Can the testis and epididymis be palpated?	Does the swelling transilluminate?	Note:
Hydrocoele	Yes	No	Yes	
Inguinal hernia	Yes	Yes	No	Cough impulse
Cord lipoma	Yes	Yes	No	Painless
Epididymal cyst	Yes	Yes	Yes	
Varicocoele	Variable	Yes	No	Bag of worms

14 Dizziness/vertigo

Box 14 gives clues about assessing a patient presenting with dizziness.

Box 14 Testing for dizziness/vertigo

Diagnosis	Duration	Tinnitus	Loss of hearing	Precipitant factors
BPPV	Seconds	None	None	Specific head movements
Ménière's disease	Hours	Unilateral	Unilateral	None
Vestibular neuronitis	Days	None	None	None
Acoustic neuroma	Varies	Unilateral, persistent	Gradual unilateral reduction	None

15 Sore throat

Sore throat has a number of causes, but Box 15 identifies the findings for various conditions.

Box 15 Some causes of sore throat

Diagnosis	General malaise and temperature	Speech	Trismus	Appearance	Neck	Bloods
Quinsy	Yes	Hot potato	Yes	Unilateral palatal swelling + uvula displacement	Enlarged nodes	↑ WCC, neutrophilia
Tonsillitis	Yes	Normal	No	Bilateral tonsil swelling + erythema ± spotty white exudate	Enlarged nodes	↑ WCC, neutrophilia
Glandular fever	Yes	Normal	No	Bilateral tonsil swelling + white membranous exudate	Massive nodes	↑ WCC, lymphocytosis Paul Bunnell test positive ↑ LFTs
Acid reflux	No	Normal	No	Normal oropharynx	Normal	Normal
Tonsil carcinoma	No	Normal	No	Unilateral tonsil swelling/ ulceration	Nodal metastases may be present	May be raised WCC

16 Dysphagia

Dysphagia has a number of causes, but Box 16 identifies the findings for various conditions.

Box 16 Some causes of dysphagia

Diagnosis	True dysphagia	Regurgitation of food	Neck swelling	Referred otalgia	Other features
Pharyngeal pouch	Yes, progressive as pouch enlarges	Yes, typically after minutes and undigested	Yes, if large	No	Diagnosis confirmed with barium swallow
Globus pharyngeus	No	No	No	No	Anxiety, lack of positive findings on examination and investigations
Hypopharyngeal carcinoma	Yes, gradually progressive from solids to liquids	If large may be regurgitation	Yes, from metastatic nodes	Yes, via IX cranial nerve	In advanced disease, may present with dysphonia secondary to vocal cord palsy
Thyroid goitre	Yes, if large	No	Antero-inferior, moves on swallowing	No	Sudden increase in size and stridor: consider malignant disease
Oesophageal achalasia	Yes, to solids and liquids	Yes	No	No	Barium swallow typically shows 'bird-beak' narrowing at gastro-oesophageal junction
Diffuse oesophageal spasm	Yes	No	No	No	Associated chest pain and corkscrew oesophagus on barium swallow
Bulbar palsy	Yes	No	No	No	Poor cough + dysphonia + dysarthria

17 Neck lumps

Box 17 identifies lumps that are likely to be implicated in EMQs.

Box 17 Some cause of neck lumps

Diagnosis	Site	Moves on swallow-ing	Moves on tongue protrusion	Other EMQ features
Thyroid swelling	Midline lower neck	Yes	No	Bruit on auscultation Signs of thyrotoxicosis (e.g. atrial fibrillation, tremor, eye signs)
Thyroglossal cyst	Typically midline region of hyoid, may be just lateral to midline	Yes	Yes	May become infected resulting in sudden increase in size and pain Transilluminates
Branchial cyst	Lateral neck just anterior to sternocleidomastoid (junction of upper third and lower two-thirds)	No	No	May present in later life with infection Position often characteristic in question
Chemodectoma	Lateral neck, bifurcation of carotid	No	No	Pulsatile and mobile laterally
Submandibular	Below ramus mandible	No	No	Bimanually palpable Stone may be palpable in submandibular duct Marginal mandibular nerve palsy in malignant cases
Parotid	Parotid region, *but* can occur at angle of mandible	No	No	VII nerve palsy in cases of malignancy
Cystic hygroma	Posterior triangle	No	No	Often young patient Brilliant transilluminance

18 The paediatric hip

These always crop up in orthopaedic EMQs and are frequently mixed up (see Box 18).

Box 18 The paediatric hip

Condition	Features
Congenital dislocation of hip	Usually detected at birth by Ortolani's/Barlow's tests May present later with delayed walking/waddling gait Extra thigh crease on examination
Perthes' disease	Usually male Hip pain and limp (3–11 years) X-ray: decreased size femoral head, patchy density
Slipped femoral epiphysis	Often obese Older than Perthes' patient (10–16 years) Groin pain, limp Flexed, abducted, externally rotated hip

19 Upper limb nerve injury

Box 19 lists clinical features of some upper limb injuries.

Box 19 Upper limb nerve injury

Nerve implicated	Features
Median nerve	Wasting at thenar eminence
	Loss of sensation, lateral palmar surface 3½ digits
	Test for weakness in abductor pollicis brevis
	Frequently affected in carpal tunnel syndrome
Ulnar nerve	Wasting at hypothenar eminence
	Sensory loss over medial 1½ fingers
	Test for weakness in abductor digiti minimi
	'Claw hand' deformity
	Positive Froment's sign
Radial nerve	Weakness of wrist extension leading to 'wrist drop'
	Anaesthesia over 1st dorsal interosseous muscle
Axillary nerve	Failure of abduction after shoulder dislocation
	Anaesthesia over military badge area of shoulder
Long thoracic nerve	Winged scapula
Klumpke's palsy (C8, T1)	Paralysis of intrinsic muscles of the hand
	Loss of sensation in ulnar distribution
	Horner's syndrome sometimes present
Erb's palsy (C5, C6)	Loss of shoulder abduction and elbow flexion
	Arm held internally rotated
	'Waiter's tip' sign if arm adducted behind back

20 Lower limb nerve injury

Box 20 lists clinical features of some lower limb injuries.

Box 20 Lower limb nerve injury

Nerve implicated	Features
Common peroneal nerve	Often a blow to lateral aspect of knee is described
	Weakness in dorsiflexion and eversion of foot
	Sensory loss over dorsum of foot
Tibial nerve	Inability to invert foot or stand on tiptoe
Sciatic nerve	Foot drop (e.g. after hip replacement)
	Sensation loss below knee, except medial lower leg (saphenous nerve)

21 Reflexes and motor nerve roots

EMQs often delineate focal weakness/loss of reflexes to identify nerve/root lesion (see Box 21).

Box 21 Nerve roots

Reflex/movement	Nerve root
Supinator	C5, C6
Biceps	C5, C6
Triceps	C7
Knee	L3, L4
Ankle	S1
Shoulder abduction	C5
Elbow flexion	C5, C6
Elbow extension	C7
Finger abduction	T1
Hip flexion	L1, L2
Hip extension	L5, S1
Knee flexion	L5, S1
Knee extension	L3, L4
Ankle dorsiflexion	L4, L5
Ankle plantar flexion	S1

22 Upper limb orthopaedic conditions

Box 22 will help in the diagnosis of conditions of the upper limb.

Box 22 Orthopaedic conditions of the upper limb

Clinical signs	Diagnosis
Thickening, fibrosis palmar fascia	Dupuytren's contracture
'Dinner fork deformity'	Colles fracture
Wrist pain on forced thumb adduction, flexion	De Quervain's syndrome
Pain, paraesthesia with median nerve distribution	Carpal tunnel syndrome
Shoulder pain on abduction 60–120°	Painful arc syndrome/supraspinatus tendonitis
Lump in upper arm after lifting	Ruptured long head of biceps
Reduced active/passive movement, stiffness of	Frozen shoulder/adhesive capsulitis shoulder

23 Lower limb orthopaedic conditions

Box 23 will help in the diagnosis of conditions of the lower limb.

Box 23 Orthopaedic conditions of the lower limb

Clinical signs	Diagnosis
Locked knee, with positive McMurray's test	Meniscal tear
Excessive anterior glide of tibia on femur	Anterior cruciate ligament tear/rupture
Typically a sport injury: non-contact deceleration with twisting in valgus position (e.g. skiing, basketball, football)	
Excessive posterior glide of tibia on femur	Posterior cruciate ligament tear/rupture
Less common: may be significant trauma pushing tibia back (e.g. against dashboard in RTA, football tackle from in front, fall on flexed knee)	
Prominent tender tibial tubercle	Osgood–Schlatter's disease
Painful soles of feet	Plantar fasciitis
Look out for associated diseases (e.g. ankylosing spondylitis)	
Elderly patient unable to weight-bear after fall	Fracture neck of femur
Shortened and externally rotated leg	
Pain over dorsum foot/metatarsal	March fracture (metatarsal)
Athlete, history of excessive walking	
Usually children/adolescents	Ewing's sarcoma
Long bones, limb girdle	
'Onion-peel' sign	
Usually adolescent	Osteosarcoma
Older peak (in patients with Paget's)	
Periosteal elevation (Codman's triangle)	

24 Red eye

The many causes of red eye are summarized in Box 24.

Box 24 Interpreting red eye

Clinical signs	Diagnosis
Blurred vision, haloes	Acute closed-angle glaucoma
Hazy cornea	
Pupil fixed and dilated	
Raised intraocular pressure	
Blurred vision, photophobia	Anterior uveitis
Inflammatory cells	
May be autoimmune disease	
Vision normal, injected conjunctiva	Bacterial conjunctivitis
Mucopurulent/lid crusting if bacterial	
Usually bilateral, watery eyes	Viral conjunctivitis
Preceding viral illness	
Follicles on conjunctiva	
Bilateral itchy eyes	Allergic conjunctivitis
History of atopy (e.g. asthma, eczema)	
History of trauma/contact lens use	Corneal ulceration
Pain, photophobia, blurred vision	
Pain, photophobia	Dendritic ulcer (HSV)
May have history of other HSV infection (e.g. cold sores)	
Fluoroscein stain: branch-like lesion	
Pain, hypopyon, ↓↓ vision	Endophthalmitis
Usually after ophthalmic surgery	

25 Retinal signs

Retinal signs are listed in Box 25.

Box 25 Interpreting retinal signs

Clinical signs	Diagnosis
Silver wiring, AV nipping, cotton wool spots, flame/dot-blot haemorrhages	Hypertensive retinopathy
Hard exudates, microaneurysms, haemorrhages, macular oedema	Diabetic retinopathy
Stormy sunset appearance	Central retinal vein occlusion
Cherry red spot at macula	Central retinal artery occlusion
Optic disc cupping	Glaucoma
Blurred, elevated disc swelling	Papilloedema
Absent venous pulsations	
Associated raised intracranial pressure	
Bone spiculing	Retinitis pigmentosa
Loss of red reflex	Cataract
'Mozzarella pizza' appearance	CMV retinitis
History of immunocompromise (e.g. HIV)	

26 Pupils

Pupilar signs are listed in Box 26.

Box 26 Interpreting pupilar signs

Clinical signs	Diagnosis
Bilateral dilated pupils	Brainstem death
Plus no vestibulo-ocular reflex	Amphetamines, cocaine
Plus euphoric	Tricyclic antidepressant overdose
Plus anticholinergic signs (e.g. ↑ pulse, ↓ BP, urinary retention)	
Bilateral pinpoint pupils	Opiate overdose
	Pontine haemorrhage
Dilated pupil	Cranial nerve III lesion
Ptosis, down-and-out pupil	Holmes–Adie pupil
Young woman, sluggish reaction to light, may have ↓ tendon reflexes	
Constricted pupil	Neurosyphilis
Irregular pupils, reacts accommodation but not light	Diabetes (Argyll Robertson pupil)
Unilateral ptosis, ipsilateral loss sweating (anhidrosis)	Horner's syndrome

27 Ocular movements

Ocular signs are listed in Box 27.

Box 27 Interpreting ocular movements

Lesion	Ocular movement
Cranial nerve III	Defective elevation, depression, adduction
Cranial nerve IV	Defective depression in adduction
	Vertical diplopia worse in down gaze
Cranial nerve VI	Failure to abduct
	Horizontal diplopia worse on abduction

28 Visual field defects

Features of visual field defects are listed in Box 28.

Box 28 Visual field defects

Clinical finding	Diagnosis
Bitemporal hemianopia	Chiasma lesion (e.g. pituitary tumour)
Superior quadrantanopia	Temporal lobe lesion
Inferior quadrantanopia	Parietal lobe lesion
Homonymous hemianopia	Optic radiation, visual cortex injury
Central scotoma	Macula (degeneration/oedema)

29 Hypertensive retinopathy

Hypertensive retinopathy is given a grading (see Box 29).

Box 29 Grading of hypertensive retinopathy

Grading	Features
I	Silver wiring
II	AV nipping
III	Grade II + haemorrhages, cotton wool spots, exudates
IV	Grade III plus papilloedema

30 Diabetic retinopathy

Retinopathy in diabetes is staged (see Box 30).

Box 30 Stages of diabetic retinopathy

Stage	Features
Background	Microaneurysms, hard exudates, flame/dot haemorrhages
Maculopathy	Background + macular retinopathy
Pre-proliferative	Maculopathy + cotton wool spots, blot haemorrhages, venous beading
Proliferative	Pre-proliferative + neovascularization of disc/retina

31 Neurosurgery/head injury

Some features of head injury likely to come up in EMQs are listed in Box 31.

Box 31 Features of head injury or pathology

Head injury or pathology	Features
Subdural haemorrhage	History of trauma
	Particularly elderly/alcoholic in EMQ
	CT: white crescentic lesion *concave* to skull
Extradural haemorrhage	Usually clear history of significant head trauma
	Lucid interval
	CT: white lesion *concave* (lentiform shape) to skull
Basal skull fracture	Anosmia, rhinorrhea
	Periorbital bruising ('raccoon eyes')
	Bruising behind ear/haemotympanum
Diffuse axonal injury	Significant head injury, comatosed but normal CT
Subarachnoid haemorrhage	Sudden-onset severe debilitating headache
	Meningism (e.g. neck stiffness)
	Lumbar puncture: xanthochromia

32 Arterial blood gases

When interpreting blood gases one should identify whether an acidosis or alkalosis is present, and then look for a metabolic or respiratory cause for the derangement and consider compensatory mechanisms. In addition to information on the patient's acid/base status, the blood gas will give information on *oxygenation, electrolyte values and glucose and lactate levels* (see Boxes 32 and 33). The normal ranges for arterial blood gases are:

- pH: 7.35–7.45

- PCO_2: 4.27–6.4 kPa

- PO_2: 11.1–14.4 kPa

- HCO_3^-: 24–28 mmol/L

- Acid/base excess (ABE): ±2

- Glucose: 3.9–5.3 mmol/L

- Lactate: 0.5–1.6 mmol/L

Box 32 Expected directional changes in blood gas results for various conditions (N, normal).

Imbalance	pH	PCO_2	HCO_3^-	ABE
Respiratory acidosis	↓	↑↑	N	N
Partially compensated	↓	↑	↑↑	↑↑
Fully compensated	N	↑	↑	↑
Respiratory alkalosis	↑	↓↓	N	N
Partially compensated	↑	↓	↓↓	↓↓
Fully compensated	N	↓	↓	↓
Metabolic acidosis	↓	N	↓↓	↓↓
Partially compensated	↓	↓↓	↓	↓
Fully compensated	N	↓	↓	↓
Metabolic alkalosis	↑	N	↑↑	↑↑
Partially compensated	↑	↑↑	↑	↑
Fully compensated	N	↑	↑	↑

33 Classical EMQ descriptions of blood gases

Box 33 Classical EMQ descriptions of blood gases

Condition	Features
Respiratory alkalosis	Anxious, hyperventilating, signs of acute hypocalcaemia
	(e.g. perioral paraesthesia, numbness, tingling)
Respiratory acidosis	Scenario with reduced respiratory effort
	(e.g. neuromuscular disease, COPD)
Metabolic acidosis	Diabetic ketoacidosis scenario, especially in undiagnosed diabetic, septic patient, renal failure
Metabolic alkalosis	Pyloric stenosis scenario in vomiting infant, purgative/laxative abuse

34 Skin cover in plastic surgery

Aspects of skin cover are listed in Box 34.

Box 34 Skin cover

Use	Type
Infected wound, cosmesis not important (e.g. post-incision and drainage of buttock abscess)	Secondary intention
Clean small wound not under tension	Primary intention
Skin cover required Can cover large areas (e.g. skin cover for burns, resurface muscle flaps) May be poor cosmesis Needs good care of donor site	Split-thickness skin graft
Smaller area skin cover Better cosmesis so good for facial defects More resistant to trauma so can use on body areas subject to abrasion	Full-thickness skin graft
Defect too large to close, or graft not possible (e.g. compound lower limb fracture) Reconstruction surgery (e.g. breast)	Flap (local/pedicled/free)

Index

pregnancy
  deep vein thrombosis 240, 244
  ectopic 35, 237, 241, 247
  proliferative diabetic retinopathy 195
  renal stones 124, 137
preoperative investigations 206, 220–1
proctocolectomy
  with ileal pouch 9, 43
  with ileostomy 9, 43
propofol 204, 217–18
propranolol 108, 113
prostate, transurethral resection 122, 133
prostate cancer 122, 126, 132,
    133–4, 140
prostate specific antigen (PSA), repeat
    122, 133–4
prostatectomy, radical 126, 133, 134,
    135, 140
Proteus 138
proximal interphalangeal joint 87, 104
psammoma body 58
pseudogout 78, 94
Pseudomonas aeruginosa 166, 167
psoriatic arthritis 77, 93
ptosis 179, 182, 189–90, 192–3
pubic ramus, fracture 82, 98
pulmonary embolism 81, 98, 210, 225,
    238, 242
pupil 179, 189–90, 272
pyloric stenosis 11, 32, 45, 72–3, 251
pyonephrosis 124, 137–8

quinsy 145, 159, 261

radial nerve injury 81, 98, 265
  axilla 90, 106
radiation therapy, external-beam 134
radiograph
  abdominal 14, 49, 237, 242
  chest 238, 242–3
  plain foot 240, 244
radiological emergencies 239, 243
radiological investigations 240, 244
radiology 236–44, 252
radius, fracture 81, 97, 99
Ramsay Hunt syndrome 149, 166
Ramstedt's procedure 32, 45, 72–3
randomized controlled trials, meta-
    analysis 33, 73–4

rectal carcinoma 8, 42, 43, 248
recurrent laryngeal nerve 163
red eye 177, 187–8, 270
red flag symptoms 35
Reed-Sternberg cells 170
reflexes 267
reflux oesophagitis 35–6
Refsum's disease 190
Reinke's oedema 163–4
Reiter's disease 77, 93
relative afferent pupillary defect 189
renal abscess 127, 142
renal calculi 34, 132, 237, 241
  associations 258
  imaging/intervention 126, 140–1
  incidence 258
  management 124, 137–8
renal cell carcinoma 119, 127, 128–9,
    141–2
renal colic 3, 34, 124, 138, 237, 241
renal cyst, simple 127, 141
renal failure 121, 132–3, 232
respiratory acidosis 211, 225, 278, 279
respiratory alkalosis 211, 278, 279
respiratory failure
  type I 199, 212, 232
  type II 199, 211–12, 228, 231–2
retinal detachment 184, 194–6
  Marcus Gunn pupil 179, 189
  Marfan syndrome 186, 196
  non-rhegmatogenous 195
  rhegmatogenous 195
retinal pigment epithelium 194–5
retinal signs 271
retinitis pigmentosa 186, 190,
    197, 271
retinoblastoma 186, 196–7
retrograde urography 140
rhabdomyolysis 129, 228, 232
rheumatoid arthritis 46, 77, 86, 92,
    102, 173
rhinitis medicamentosa 146, 162
rhinorrhoea 28, 67
rhinosinusitis 161
rib
  cervical 151, 169
  fracture 239, 243
Rigler's sign 243
ryanodine receptor defects 225